High-Yield™

Surgery

SECOND EDITION

High-Yield™

Surgery

SECOND EDITION

R. Nirula, MD
Assistant Professor of Surgery
Medical College of Wisconsin
Department of Surgery, Division of Trauma/Critical Care
Milwaukee, Wisconsin

LIPPINCOTT WILLIAMS & WILKINS
A **Wolters Kluwer** Company
Philadelphia • Baltimore • New York • London
Buenos Aires • Hong Kong • Sydney • Tokyo

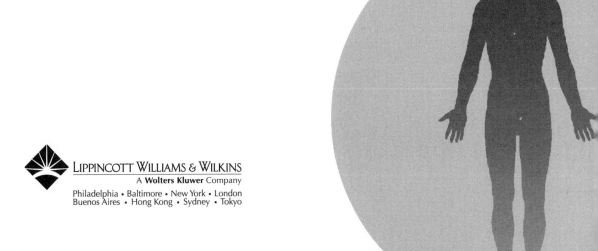

Acquisitions Editor: Donna Balado
Managing Editor: Tenille Sands
Marketing Manager: Emilie Linkins
Production Editor: Jennifer Ajello
Designer: Terry Mallon
Compositor: Circle Graphics
Printer: Courier-Kendallville

Library of Congress Cataloging-in-Publication Data

Nirula, R. (Raminder)
   High-yield surgery / R. Nirula.—2nd ed.
      p. ; cm.
   Includes index.
   ISBN 0-7817-7656-2
      1. Surgery—Outlines, syllabi, etc. 2. Surgery—Decision making—Outlines, syllabi, etc. I.
Title.
   [DNLM: 1. Surgical Procedures, Operative—methods—Outlines. 2. Decision Making—Outlines.
WO 18.2 N721h 2005]
   RD31.5N55 2005
   617—dc22

                                                                              2005049440

Contents

Chapter 1

Preoperative, Perioperative, and Postoperative Considerations

I Surgical Risk Assessment

Patients undergoing surgery must be assessed for their perioperative risk for both the specific procedure and the general anesthetic agent. Specific diseases should alert the physician to the need for further preoperative workup or modifications in the postoperative management. Particular attention should be paid to (1) diabetes mellitus, (2) renal function, (3) cardiac function, (4) liver function, (5) pulmonary function, and (6) thromboembolism risk.

A. DIABETES MELLITUS

1. **Preoperative assessment**
   a. The patient should be assessed for signs and symptoms of long-standing diabetes, including neuropathy, nephropathy, peripheral vascular disorders, and cardiac disease.
   b. Laboratory assessment should include tests for serum glucose, hemoglobin A_{1C}, and serum creatinine.
   c. A preoperative electrocardiogram should be performed, even if the patient denies a history of myocardial infarction, because patients with diabetes have an increased incidence of silent myocardial infarction.

2. **Perioperative management**
   a. The patient's blood glucose level should be well controlled (125–180 mg/dL) before operation.
   b. Intraoperative blood glucose monitoring is necessary for major procedures on patients who take insulin. If the blood glucose level becomes elevated, treatment with short-acting insulin is necessary.
   c. For **minor procedures**, if the patient did not eat breakfast, morning hypoglycemic agents should be withheld. The patient should be treated as necessary with short-acting insulin. After surgery, the patient should return to the normal regimen once normal eating resumes.
   d. For patients with diabetes who need **total parenteral nutrition (TPN)**, insulin infusions may be necessary to maintain glucose homeostasis. These infusions can be administered as a separate drip given intravenously or they can be added to the TPN bag. If the blood glucose level is difficult to control, neutral protamine Hagedorn insulin can be administered to reduce the intravenous drip requirements. Fingerstick blood sugar measurements should be obtained every 4–6 hours.
   e. Once patients are receiving a diabetic diet, they can be returned to their preoperative insulin or oral hypoglycemic regimen.
   f. Adequate hydration to prevent prerenal azotemia is essential. These patients often have some baseline renal impairment that can be worsened by perioperative fluid shifts.

B. RENAL FUNCTION
1. Preoperative assessment
    a. Patients who have known renal failure and receive routine dialysis should have their electrolytes, blood urea nitrogen (BUN), and creatinine measured before surgery. Particular attention should be paid to potassium. Extra potassium should not be administered intravenously unless abnormally low values are present (unlikely).

    b. Volume status should be assessed, and the need for dialysis secondary to volume overload should be determined. Jugular venous distension, signs of pulmonary edema, and changes in daily weights are useful in this case.

    c. Hypertension, cardiac disease, and diabetes often coexist in patients who have renal insufficiency. Appropriate workup should be performed.

2. Perioperative management
    a. Bleeding times are often elevated as a result of uremia-induced platelet dysfunction. Patients who are undergoing major procedures may need vasopressin to partially correct this abnormality.

    b. In the acute setting, volume overload, acidosis, and hyperkalemia must be corrected by dialysis to reduce perioperative mortality.

    c. Patients who are hyperkalemic but do not need dialysis immediately before surgery may be given sodium polystyrene sulfonate (Kayexalate) orally or rectally to bind potassium and lower serum potassium levels over several hours.

    d. Patients who have electrocardiogram (EKG) changes or rising potassium levels (usually >6 or 7 mg/dL) should receive insulin and glucose or calcium intravenously to drive potassium into the cells.

    e. Pancuronium, tubocurarine (neuromuscular blockers that potentiate hyperkalemia), gallamine (excreted by the kidneys and not dialyzable), and methoxyflurane (nephrotoxic) are contraindicated anesthetic agents.

    f. Hypotension should be avoided to prevent thrombosis of arteriovenous fistulas that are used for dialysis.

    g. Fluids, electrolytes, and pH should be monitored closely postoperatively with low-maintenance, low-sodium intravenous fluids.

    h. Patients who are undergoing major procedures with bowel anastomosis and are nutritionally deprived should not receive the low-protein diets routinely given to patients with renal disease. A high-calorie diet with adequate protein should be instituted to improve healing and immune function. If necessary, the frequency of dialysis should be increased to combat the elevated urea that results from increased protein intake.

    i. Most patients with renal failure are anemic. Therefore, administration of packed red cells may be necessary with moderate blood loss.

C. CARDIAC FUNCTION
1. Preoperative assessment
    a. Patients who are younger than 45 years of age and have no history of coronary artery disease and no cardiac symptoms can usually undergo major procedures without preoperative cardiac workup.

    b. Patients who have symptoms of congestive heart failure (CHF), angina, dyspnea, or syncope or have a history of myocardial infarction require preoperative EKG and chest radiograph.

    c. Patients who have a history of dysrhythmia should undergo 24-hour monitoring and appropriate treatment preoperatively.

    d. Subsequent workup involves an exercise EKG (stress test). This test shows ST-segment depression in people with significant coronary artery disease. If ST-segment depression occurs, a coronary angiogram should be obtained and pre-operative medical management, angioplasty, or coronary artery bypass grafting should be considered.

e. Patients who have poor exercise tolerance unrelated to cardiac disease should undergo a stress thallium scan with a coronary vasodilator (e.g., dipyridamole). The radioisotope (thallium) will distribute into the myocardium that is perfused by normal vessels but will not be taken up by the myocardium that is supplied by diseased vessels.

f. Patients who have a history of CHF should have an echocardiogram to determine the left ventricular function and detect valvular disease. Patients who have valvular heart disease have narrow limits of optimal cardiac function with respect to intravascular volume status. Too little volume results in hypotension, and too much results in overload.

g. The risk of cardiac-related mortality in noncardiac surgical patients is assessed using several factors (Table 1-1). Patients with fewer than 6 points have a 1% mortality risk. Those with 6–12 points have a 5% mortality risk. Those with 13–25 points have an 11% mortality risk. Those with more than 25 points have a 22% mortality risk.

2. **Perioperative management**

a. Patients who have significant coronary artery disease and are undergoing **emergent noncardiac surgery** should be monitored with a pulmonary artery catheter and an arterial line. This monitoring permits tight intravascular volume control based on pulmonary wedge pressure. It also monitors changes in cardiac output, which can reflect the need for inotropic support (i.e., dopamine, dobutamine, phosphodiesterase inhibitors, or epinephrine), versus beta blockade to reduce myocardial oxygen demands.

b. In patients who have significant cardiac disease that is managed medically and are undergoing **elective major procedures**, the risk of perioperative myocardial infarction can be reduced with tight intravascular volume control. Reduction of afterload is also needed in those who have hypertension. Afterload reduction can be accomplished by preoperative placement of a pulmonary artery catheter

TABLE 1-1	CARDIAC RISK INDEX
Risk Factor	**Points**
S3 heart sound, CHF, or JVD	11
Recent myocardial infarction (<6 months ago)	10
Dysrhythmia	7
Age >70 years	5
Emergency operation	4
PaO_2 <60 mm Hg	3
$PaCO_2$ >50 mm Hg	3
Potassium <3 mEq/L	3
BUN >50 mg/dL	3
Creatinine >3 mg/dL	3
Aortic stenosis	3
Intrathoracic operation	3
Intraabdominal operation	3
Aortic operation	3

BUN = blood urea nitrogen; CHF = congestive heart failure; JVD = jugular venous distension; PaO_2 = partial pressure of oxygen in arteries; $PaCO_2$ = partial pressure of carbon dioxide in arteries.

and an arterial line. If fluid overload is present before surgery, diuretics should be administered. If the patient is hypovolemic, then fluid should be administered. General anesthesia causes vasodilation and reduces coronary artery blood flow, increasing the risk of infarction. For most people, a pulmonary artery pressure of 12–18 mm Hg is optimal.

c. In general, perioperative beta blockade can reduce the incidence of myocardial infarction in appropriately selected patients. A pulmonary artery catheter must be used because the negative inotropic effects can cause CHF if intravascular fluid volume is not appropriately managed.

d. Changes in the ST segments during anesthesia, dysrhythmias, or a drop in measured cardiac output indicates a possible myocardial infarction or ischemia. In these cases, EKG and measurement of cardiac enzymes should be performed postoperatively to determine whether infarction has occurred. These patients should be monitored in the intensive care unit and should be considered for emergent cardiac catheterization and angioplasty versus coronary artery bypass grafting. Myocardial oxygen demands must be minimized by reducing tachycardia and afterload and avoiding fluid overload.

D. LIVER FUNCTION

1. **Preoperative assessment.** Liver dysfunction significantly increases perioperative mortality. Therefore, only necessary surgical procedures should be undertaken in affected patients. The **Child's criteria** define the degree of hepatic dysfunction with respect to mortality risk (Table 1-2).

a. Patients undergoing surgery should be assessed with respect to their volume status because their intravascular volume is often depleted in the presence of significant ascites. These patients are at risk for renal failure perioperatively as well as for subsequent hepatorenal syndrome, which carries a high mortality rate.

b. Risk of bleeding is often increased, so prothrombin time (PT) and partial thromboplastin time (PTT) should be checked. These are often prolonged because of decreased production of coagulation factors by the diseased liver.

c. Anemia is often present. Therefore, the patient's hemoglobin status and the need for transfusion should be assessed.

d. Hypokalemia may be present. Therefore, the patient's potassium level should be checked.

e. The degree of ascites may lead to poor pulmonary function postoperatively because of increased abdominal distension. A therapeutic paracentesis may be useful.

f. Encephalopathy may occur perioperatively as a result of drugs, volume depletion, electrolyte disturbance, and constipation. Ammonium levels also may be elevated and may lead to encephalopathy.

TABLE 1-2	CHILD'S CRITERIA FOR HEPATIC DYSFUNCTION AND RELATED PERIOPERATIVE MORTALITY				
Classification (Risk)	Serum Bilirubin (mg/dL)	Serum Albumin (g/dL)	Ascites	Neurologic Status	Nutrition
A (minimal)	<2.0	>3.5	None	Normal	Excellent
B (moderate)	2.0–3.0	3.0–3.5	Easily controlled	Mild cognitive deficits	Good
C (high)	>3.0	<3.0	Poorly controlled	Severe deficits/coma	Wasting

g. Malnutrition is often present and is indicated by retinol-binding protein, albumin, and prealbumin levels.

2. **Perioperative management**
   a. If volume status is difficult to determine or manage, a pulmonary artery catheter should be placed preoperatively.
   b. All electrolyte disturbances should be corrected preoperatively.
   c. Patients who have a recent history of constipation and who have elevated ammonium levels should receive a form of laxative or lactulose to reduce the risk of encephalopathy.
   d. Patients whose nutritional status is poor should receive enteral feeding supplementation, or TPN that is rich in branch-chained amino acids (e.g., leucine, isoleucine, valine) and low in aromatic amino acids (e.g., tyrosine, phenylalanine) should be administered. High amounts of aromatic amino acids increase the risk of encephalopathy.
   e. Coagulopathy should be treated preoperatively with the administration of fresh-frozen plasma (FFP) and vitamin K.

E. **PULMONARY FUNCTION**
   1. **Preoperative assessment**
      a. Patients who have a history of exercise intolerance, dyspnea, wheezing, smoking, cough, or sputum production should be evaluated before any elective major operation.
      b. Patients who have small airway or chronic obstructive pulmonary disease (COPD) should have spirometry studies. A forced expiratory volume per 1 second (FEV_1) that is less than 70% of the expected value indicates obstructive airway disease or bronchospasm. A forced vital capacity that is less than 50% of the expected value for the patient's size and weight is associated with an increased incidence of postoperative complications.
      c. Arterial blood gas should be measured in patients who have major pulmonary dysfunction. This measurement provides a baseline for comparison with postoperative changes. A partial pressure of carbon dioxide higher than 45 mm Hg indicates significant alveolar hypoventilation.
      d. Patients undergoing lung resection must be assessed for their ability to tolerate lung removal postoperatively. Patients undergoing pneumonectomy should have an FEV_1 greater than 2 L preoperatively. If they do not, ventilation–perfusion studies should be obtained to quantify the degree to which the reduced ventilatory function is caused by removal of the affected lung.
      e. Patients who are malnourished are at increased risk for perioperative pneumonia. Therefore, albumin, prealbumin, or retinol-binding protein levels should be determined in patients with chronic illness and those who have a history of poor dietary intake.
      f. A chest radiograph should be obtained in patients who have a history of lung disease and those with abnormal findings on pulmonary function studies or arterial blood gas studies. The chest radiograph may identify patients whose pulmonary dysfunction is caused by COPD, pneumonia, atelectasis, effusions, or cardiac etiologies.
   2. **Perioperative management**
      a. Patients who have suboptimal pulmonary function should be instructed preoperatively to use an incentive spirometer to strengthen their respiratory muscles.
      b. Patients who have small airway disease should undergo repeat pulmonary function studies after bronchodilator therapy. If improvement occurs, patients should receive bronchodilator therapy preoperatively and postoperatively.

c. Smokers should stop smoking preoperatively.

d. Before any elective operation, patients with chronic bronchitis or pneumonia who have sputum that is positive for an organism should be treated with antibiotics until the infection resolves.

e. Optimal pain management is crucial to permit maximal lung expansion. In some cases, an epidural anesthetic is necessary postoperatively.

f. Incentive spirometry should be instituted once the patient awakens from anesthesia to reduce postoperative atelectasis and pneumonia. Early mobilization of the patient reduces ventilation–perfusion mismatch and improves lung expansion.

g. Patients who have severe COPD may need steroid therapy in addition to inhalation bronchodilators.

F. THROMBOEMBOLISM RISK

1. Preoperative assessment

a. **Virchow's triad** (i.e., venous stasis, endothelial damage, and hypercoagulability) predisposes patients to the formation of deep vein thrombosis. The subsequent risk is the development of pulmonary embolism, which can be fatal.

b. **Increased risk factors** for deep vein thrombosis include major operation, general anesthesia, obesity, age older than 70 years, malignancy, hypercoagulation disorder (protein C and S deficiency or antithrombin III deficiency), trauma, and sepsis.

c. Patients who have a history of deep vein thrombosis should undergo a hypercoagulability workup (see I F 1 b).

d. Many patients with deep vein thrombosis do not have leg swelling, edema, or pain in the calf. Their absence should not deter the clinician from further evaluation if deep vein thrombosis is suspected.

e. Duplex ultrasonography of the femoral venous system is used to determine the presence of deep vein thrombosis. This technique may also infer the presence of pelvic vein thrombus based on changes in pressures in the femoral venous system.

2. Perioperative management

a. All patients undergoing a major procedure with general anesthesia should wear leg compression devices to reduce the risk of deep vein thrombosis. These devices should be working before the induction of general anesthetic because these agents increase venous stasis. Leg compression devices should be used postoperatively until the patient is ambulating.

b. Patients who are at increased risk should receive subcutaneous heparin or low–molecular-weight heparin before and after surgery until they are ambulating.

c. Patients who have a hypercoagulable disorder require a consultation with a hematologist to manage their anticoagulation in the perioperative period and minimize the risk of deep vein thrombosis and hemorrhage.

d. Once a deep vein thrombosis is found, systemic heparinization or high-dose low–molecular-weight heparin followed by warfarin therapy should be instituted to reduce the risk of extension and subsequent embolism. If anticoagulation is contraindicated, a vena cava filter should be placed.

Ⅱ Fluid and Electrolytes

A. COMPOSITION AND DISTRIBUTION OF BODY FLUIDS

1. Total body water, which is two-thirds intracellular fluid and one-third extracellular fluid, comprises 50%–60% of a person's body mass. The extracellular fluid volume is subdivided into interstitial fluid, which is 80% of the extracellular fluid volume, and intravascular fluid, which is 20% of the extracellular fluid volume.

2. The composition of the **interstitial fluid** is similar to that of the intravascular fluid, except that the interstitial fluid contains less protein. Sodium is the predominant cation, and there are small amounts of potassium, calcium, and magnesium.

3. **Intracellular fluid** has magnesium and potassium as the main cations and low amounts of sodium.

4. **Gastric secretions** are usually hypotonic. The sodium chloride content is 75–100 mEq/L. Pancreatic and bile secretions are similar and are more isotonic. The sodium chloride content is 120–140 mEq/L. Pancreatic secretions are high in bicarbonate (approximately 100 mEq/L). Proximal small bowel fluid is nearly isotonic, but distal small bowel fluid is hypotonic.

5. Losses of gastric and distal small bowel fluid should be replaced with a hypotonic solution (e.g., 0.45% NaCl). Pancreatic and duodenal losses should be replaced with lactated Ringer's solution.

B. VOLUME DEPLETION AND VOLUME EXCESS

1. Volume depletion

    a. **Signs of intravascular volume depletion** include dry mucous membranes, decreased tissue turgor, decreased urine output, tachycardia, and hypotension. These may be present in varying degrees depending on the degree of depletion.

    b. **Laboratory indicators of hypovolemia** include a high urine specific gravity, a low urine sodium content, an elevated BUN:creatinine ratio (. 20) and a rising hematocrit value.

    c. The **goals of volume repletion** are to achieve normal circulating blood volume, as evidenced by a return to normal vital signs and urine output greater than 0.5 mL/kg/hr. If the patient is bleeding, blood should be replaced and the source of bleeding identified and stopped. Other fluid losses should be replaced as described earlier. Standard replacement fluid should be isotonic (e.g., lactated Ringer's solution). Albumin can be used in patients who have decreased oncotic pressure.

    d. In patients who have a history of cardiac disease, replenishing volume without producing fluid overload may be difficult. A pulmonary artery catheter may be required to determine intravascular volume and the need for further replacement.

2. Volume excess

    a. **Signs of intravascular volume overload** may include CHF, anasarca, and hepatomegaly. This condition may cause hypoxia, tachypnea, and tachycardia. A decrease in hematocrit also may be present.

    b. Management involves reducing intravenous fluid administration and administering furosemide if pulmonary edema is present.

C. SODIUM AND POTASSIUM IMBALANCE

1. **Hyponatremia** may occur because of hyperglycemia (pseudohyponatremia), administration of hypotonic solution, or excess diuretics in surgical patients. Mild hyponatremia can be treated by replacing losses with isotonic solution, restricting free-water intake, and correcting hyperglycemia when present.

2. **Hypernatremia** results from decreased free water intake or excess free water loss. For every 3-mEq/L elevation in serum sodium higher than 140 mEq/L, there is a free water deficit of approximately 1 L. Half of the volume should be given in the first 12 hours, and the remainder over the next 24–48 hours. The serum sodium should not be corrected too quickly (it should not decrease more than 10 mEq/L in a 6-hour period) because this will cause significant cerebral fluid accumulation and edema.

3. **Hypokalemia** may result from gastrointestinal losses, cellular shifts of potassium into the cell with hydrogen out of the cell in alkalosis, or diuresis. Persistent hypomagnesemia reduces the ability of the kidney to reabsorb potassium and makes hypokalemia difficult to correct. Dysrhythmias are the major concern with hypokalemia. Potassium losses are replaced in doses of 10 mEq/hr. Underlying alkalosis and hypomagnesemia must be corrected.

4. **Hyperkalemia** may result from overadministration of potassium, tissue injury with cellular release, renal failure, or cellular shifts during acidosis. Dysrhythmias are the major concern. Treatment involves the use of intravenous solutions without potassium. If increased potassium levels are associated with EKG changes (i.e., peaked T waves, widening QRS) or levels are greater than 7.5 mEq/L, then 10 mL 10% calcium gluconate given over a 5-minute period can reduce electrical cardiac excitability. If EKG changes are minor or potassium levels are between 6.5 and 7.5 mEq/L, **insulin** and dextrose should be administered. For milder hyperkalemia, polystyrene sulfonate (Kayexalate) binds intestinal potassium to reduce absorption.

III Surgical Bleeding and Transfusions

Evaluation and treatment of the patient who is bleeding postoperatively requires an understanding of the hemostatic process, the causes of surgical bleeding, and transfusion therapy.

A. HEMOSTASIS. Initial hemostasis begins with vasoconstriction followed by the formation of a platelet plug. An initial white thrombus is formed and is stabilized by activation of the extrinsic and intrinsic clotting cascades (Figure 1-1).

1. Preoperative patients should be questioned about abnormal bleeding with dental procedures, previous surgeries, or minor trauma; easy bruising; and family history of excessive bleeding. Screening tests (e.g., platelet count, PT, PTT) should be performed in patients who have a positive history or those undergoing a major procedure that causes significant blood loss.

2. Patients who have **normal PT, PTT**, and **platelet counts** but who exhibit **abnormal bleeding tendencies** should undergo a bleeding time test. This test assesses the functional ability of the platelets. Prolonged bleeding times are seen in patients with renal failure and those undergoing therapy with aspirin or nonsteroidal anti-inflammatory

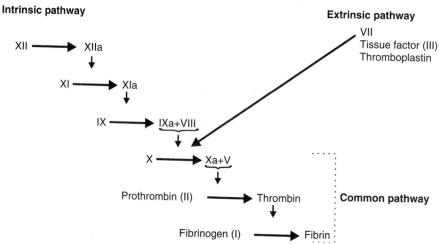

● **Figure 1.1** Coagulation pathways.

drugs (NSAIDs). Platelet disorders (e.g., von Willebrand's disease) and qualitative platelet defects cause prolonged bleeding time. All patients who take NSAIDs or aspirin should stop taking these medications 7–10 days before surgery because the effects on platelets are irreversible. This ensures sufficient time for the formation of new platelets with normal function.

3. An **elevated PT** indicates a defect in the extrinsic or common pathway. This defect indicates a deficiency in factor VII, X, V, II, or I. This value is usually elevated in patients who receive warfarin therapy.

4. An **elevated PTT** indicates a defect in the intrinsic and common pathways. This defect may indicate a deficiency in factor XII, XI, IX, VIII, X, V, II, or I. This test is useful in assessing the adequacy of heparin anticoagulation.

5. **Prolonged thrombin time** indicates a lack of conversion of fibrinogen to fibrin after the administration of thrombin. Elevated thrombin time is seen in patients with disseminated intravascular coagulation (DIC) when fibrin-split products and hypo-fibrinogenemia are present, those receiving heparin therapy, and those with dysfunctional fibrin.

B. **CAUSES OF SURGICAL BLEEDING.** Patients who have normal coagulation function preoperatively may bleed postoperatively for several reasons, including:
1. Inadequate surgical hemostasis
2. Hypothermia (decreases clotting factor function)
3. Circulating heparin administered during surgery
4. DIC, which is caused by abnormal intravascular activation of the clotting cascade and consumes enough coagulation factors to produce bleeding
5. Dilutional coagulopathy because of multiple transfusions of packed cells without replenishment of platelets and clotting factors (usually after transfusion of 6 units)

C. **TRANSFUSION THERAPY**
1. In most patients who undergo procedures that cause significant blood loss, the postoperative hemoglobin level should be maintained at approximately 10 mg/dL. This level provides an optimal ratio of oxygen-carrying capacity and decreased viscosity to facilitate circulation in the microvasculature. Younger patients may be able to tolerate a lower hemoglobin level. If tachycardia, hypotension, or active coronary artery disease are not present, a hemoglobin level as low as 7.0 mg/dL may be acceptable.

2. In the emergent life-threatening setting, patients should receive O-negative blood while blood is being crossmatched. Otherwise, type-specific blood should be used in the semi-emergent setting (10–15 minutes required). Crossmatched blood should be used in the stable patient (45 minutes required).

3. **Complications of blood transfusion** include hemolytic reaction as a result of incompatibility, fever, HIV (risk = 1/500,000), hepatitis B (risk = 1/60,000), and hepatitis C (risk = 1/30,000). Patients with fever can be treated with antipyretics and observed. Those with a hemolytic reaction have tachycardia and hypotension. In this case, the transfusion must be stopped and rechecked along with the crossmatching process. Aggressive hemodynamic support is needed to prevent renal dysfunction. DIC must be managed aggressively with replenishment of coagulation factors as indicated.

4. Transfusion of platelets is required preoperatively if the platelet count is less than 100,000/mL. Postoperatively, if there is ongoing bleeding, platelets should be transfused to maintain a count higher than 100,000/mL. If there is no active bleeding, platelet counts higher than 20,000/mL are permissible. Lower counts are associated with spontaneous bleeding.

5. Patients with elevated PT or PTT should FFP if active bleeding is present. The levels should be rechecked after administration of FFP (usually 1–2 units). The process should be repeated until normal values are attained or bleeding ceases. Occasionally, PT or PTT levels are not corrected with FFP, and a circulating anticoagulant must be considered. Also, factor VIII levels are low in FFP. Therefore, in patients who have significant dilutional coagulopathy, cryoprecipitate, which is rich in factor VIII, should be administered.

6. Patients who have specific factor deficiencies should receive these factors preoperatively and postoperatively for several days.

Ⓘⓥ Infection Control

A. **THE NEED FOR PERIOPERATIVE ANTIBIOTICS** is based on the risk of contamination during the surgical procedure.

1. **Clean cases** do not involve contamination from endogenous flora and involve surgical sites that are uncontaminated at the time of surgery. Examples include breast surgery, hernia repair, and thyroidectomy. In these cases, preoperative antibiotics are not required because there is little reduction in perioperative wound infection when adequate aseptic technique is used.

2. **Clean-contaminated cases** involve entry into a surgical field that is initially clean, with entry into a colonized area during the operation. Examples include elective colon resection, elective gastric or small bowel surgery, and common bile duct exploration. In general, perioperative antibiotics started before induction and continued for up to 24 hours postoperatively are indicated. The antibiotics should include gram-negative and anaerobic coverage for intestinal surgery. Usually, a second-generation cephalosporin is adequate.

3. **Dirty cases** involve an established infection, such as a perforated viscus or an infarcted bowel. These cases have a high postoperative infection rate. Antibiotics are started preoperatively and considered postoperatively for more than 24 hours.

4. **Procedures that involve the implantation of a prosthesis** and patients who have a prosthetic in place (e.g., heart valve, vascular graft) require adequate gram-positive coverage during clean cases. The result of a prosthetic infection may be catastrophic. Usually, a first-generation cephalosporin is adequate.

B. **COMMON POSTOPERATIVE INFECTIONS** include pneumonia, urinary tract infections, and central venous catheter infections. These should be managed as they appear. Early mobilization and removal of a Foley catheter and intravenous lines when no longer necessary can reduce the incidence of these infections.

1. Patients who receive long-term antibiotics, immunocompromised patients, and those who receive TPN have an increased risk of fungal infection (*Candida*). Usually, these patients have fever, with or without leukocytosis, and respond to antifungal treatment (fluconazole).

2. Patients who undergo elective colon resection should have a mechanical bowel preparation, oral antibiotics, and intravenous antibiotics preoperatively to cover gram-negative and anaerobic organisms. This approach drastically reduces perioperative infection rates.

3. In patients who have gross spillage from a perforated viscus or gross intra-abdominal infection, the skin wound should be left open because the risk of wound infection is so high. This allows the wound to heal by secondary intention without the development of wound abscess, which can prolong the hospital course and cause sepsis.

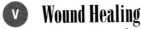

Wound Healing

Healing occurs by the following mechanisms: (1) **Primary wound healing** occurs when the wound is closed by direct approximation of the wound edges. (2) **Secondary wound healing** occurs when the wound is left open to granulate, contract, and heal on its own, without suture closure. (3) **Tertiary wound closure** is delayed apposition of the wound edges after infection in the wound subsides and the wound begins to granulate.

A. After tissue injury, small vessels contract. Platelets are deposited, and the clotting cascade is activated. Platelets and damaged endothelial cells release chemotactic factors and factors that increase permeability and perfusion to the wound site, leading to subsequent hyperemia. This is the beginning of the first phase of wound healing: the **inflammatory phase.**

B. **Neutrophils** migrate to the site and attach to the endothelium that migrates into the wound. They are the predominant cells in the first 48 hours after injury. These cells secrete chemotactic substances as well as complement and kallikrein. They act against offending organisms but are not crucial for wound healing to complete. The neutropenic patient has a higher incidence of wound infections, but the wounds will still heal to completion if they are not infected.

C. **Macrophages** predominate after the first 24–48 hours and secrete macrophage-derived growth factor and wound angiogenesis factor. The result is fibroblast proliferation and the development of new blood vessels. These cells are crucial to the eventual healing of wounds.

D. Once epithelium grows over the wound, the **proliferative phase** begins, usually by day 3 or 4. Fibroblasts prevail and begin to manufacture collagen, which requires adequate vitamin C stores for the hydroxylation of proline and lysine. The collagen fibrils are woven into a helix and secreted into the wound matrix.

E. The secreted collagen is known as **procollagen.** The procollagen has several terminal amino acids removed, creating **tropocollagen.** Tropocollagen molecules link to form the final collagen matrix.

F. The final phase is the **maturation phase.** This phase involves collagen remodeling over several months.

Surgical Nutrition

Poor perioperative surgical nutrition leads to increased morbidity and mortality.

A. Patients with a **recent weight loss of 10% or more** can have a significantly increased rate of complications, including pneumonia, wound infection, anastomotic breakdown, and septic complications. In general, healthy patients undergoing elective surgery with a normal nutritional status can tolerate supplementation with only 5% dextrose intravenous solution for 5–8 days. After that, if enteral nutrition can be instituted, hyperalimentation should be implemented.

B. In the patient who is undergoing elective surgery, **body weight** may indicate undernutrition or overnutrition compared with the ideal weight for a given height. In patients with significant illness, body weight may be changed as a result of changes in body water.

These changes do not correlate with overall nutritional status. For this reason, body weight is less useful in predicting the need for supplementation.

C. **Low serum albumin levels** are seen in malnourished patients. However, in ill patients, hypoalbuminemia may be caused by several factors that are unrelated to nutritional status. Therefore, albumin levels are less specific than other measures of adequate nutrition. Further, albumin levels change over 1–2 weeks in response to increases in nutrition, so albumin level is a delayed indicator of changing nutritional status.

D. **Prealbumin** is a transport protein for thyroid hormones. It has a more rapid turnover (2–3 days) than albumin. Sepsis, trauma, and renal function affect prealbumin levels regardless of nutritional status, limiting its specificity.

E. **Poor hand grip and respiratory muscle strength** indicates diminished nutritional status. These findings correlate well with postoperative complications.

F. Patients who cannot take adequate enteral nutrition before elective surgery should receive **TPN** until their nutritional status improves. TPN is particularly important in patients undergoing intestinal anastomosis because inadequate nutrition increases the risk of anastomotic leak.

VII Postoperative Infection

The incidence of postoperative infection depends on the patient's nutritional status, immune function, and comorbid conditions as well as on the surgical technique, degree of contamination, and perioperative prophylaxis.

A. The patient who undergoes a **major abdominal or thoracic operation** is at risk for postoperative pneumonia. These patients have reduced total lung capacity secondary to atelectasis from pain and immobility. Poor clearance of secretions and reduced lung expansion leads to plugging of the airways and subsequent infection with nosocomial bacteria. These patients are also at risk for aspiration pneumonia, especially when they are oversedated. Most cases of postoperative pneumonia are caused by gram-negative organisms. Fungal pneumonia may occur in immunocompromised patients.
   1. **Symptoms.** Typically, fever and sputum production are noted after the third or fourth postoperative day. Patients may have a rising white cell count, and a chest radiograph usually shows bilateral atelectasis and infiltrate.
   2. **Treatment.** Coverage with a third-generation cephalosporin, improved pulmonary aeration, and sputum culture are required.

B. Patients with a **Foley catheter** are at risk for urinary tract infection.
   1. **Symptoms.** Urinary tract infections typically evolve after the first 3–4 days postoperatively. Patients have irritation from the catheter and may have a low-grade fever. Urinalysis shows leukocytes or nitrates as well as white blood cells. A culture usually grows gram-negative organisms. In immunocompromised patients, fungal organisms may appear.
   2. **Treatment.** Adequate treatment involves removal of the catheter when possible and appropriate antibiotic coverage with a fluoroquinolone or second-generation cephalosporin.

C. **Wound infection** usually occurs 4–5 days after surgery. Necrotizing *Clostridium* infection can occur within 24–48 hours.

1. **Symptoms.** Patients usually have a low-grade fever as well as redness and pain at the wound site. The wound should be squeezed to express pus.
2. **Treatment.** If no fluctuance or pus is noted, then the diagnosis is cellulitis. It can be managed with a first-generation cephalosporin because it is usually caused by a gram-positive organism. Infections after bowel surgery are usually gram-negative or anaerobic and are often associated with abscess formation. In these cases, the wound must be opened to allow adequate drainage. This therapy is often adequate, but most clinicians also use antibiotics against gram-negative and anaerobic organisms.

D. **Intra-abdominal infections** may result from dehiscence of a gastrointestinal anastomosis or formation of an abscess secondary to the initial disease process, necessitating surgery.
1. **Symptoms.** For example, a patient with a perforated appendix undergoes an appendectomy. On the fourth postoperative day, the patient still has no bowel function. The abdomen is distended and tender, and the temperature and white cell count are elevated. This patient most likely has a pelvic abscess caused by the initial contamination of the perforated appendix.
2. **Treatment.** Computed tomography–guided drainage of the abdominal abscess is often successful and acquires material for culture. Antibiotics against gram-negative organisms, enterococci, and anaerobes are necessary. Patients who have an anastomotic breakdown need emergent reoperation to fix the problem as well as antibiotics and significant resuscitation.

E. **Line sepsis** usually occurs after a central line has been in place for more than 5–7 days.
1. **Symptoms.** Patients have fever spikes or a rising white cell count. Usually, removal of the line and culture of the tip establishes the diagnosis. Antibiotics are not usually required once the line is removed. Thrombophlebitis can occur at the peripheral intravenous site and can be prevented by changing the intravenous site every 3 days.
2. **Treatment.** If a palpable cord is present at the site, the infected vein should be resected under local anesthetic. Organisms responsible are typically gram positive. If necessary, a first-generation cephalosporin, penicillin, or vancomycin may be used.

Chapter 2

Esophageal Disorders

Motility Disorders

A. ACHALASIA

1. **General characteristics**
   a. Failure of esophageal body peristalsis occurs when there is incomplete relaxation of the lower esophageal sphincter (LES).
   b. Achalasia may be caused by neuronal degeneration of the esophageal myenteric plexus, an infiltrating tumor of the cardia of the stomach, or a tight Nissen fundoplication.
   c. Achalasia also occurs in patients who have scleroderma.

2. **Clinical features** include:
   a. Dysphagia
   b. Regurgitation, which is different from vomiting in that the material has little or no sour or bitter taste (as noted with gastric contents)
   c. Chest pain with no significant findings on cardiac workup
   d. Weight loss over time as a result of decreased caloric intake
   e. Microaspiration, which may cause pulmonary dysfunction and chronic cough

3. **Diagnosis**
   a. **Esophageal dilation** with an air–fluid level shown on a plain upright chest radiograph indicates an aperistaltic or obstructed esophagus.
   b. **Barium swallow** shows the dilated esophagus. The distal esophagus typically has a narrowed, **"bird beak" appearance** (Figure 2-1).
   c. **Endoscopy** is performed to look at the cardia of the stomach to rule out tumor.
   d. **Manometry** establishes the diagnosis and shows elevated LES pressure with incomplete relaxation and absence of esophageal body peristalsis.

4. **Treatment**
   a. **Balloon dilation** is performed endoscopically. However, this procedure carries a risk of esophageal perforation, which can be life-threatening. The success rate is 60%–70%.
   b. If balloon dilation is unsuccessful, the **Heller myotomy** procedure (division of the circular muscle of the lower esophagus) should be performed. An antireflux procedure must also be performed. Hemifundoplication is used because a full Nissen fundoplication causes dysphagia and prevents the transit of food past the wrap. During the procedure, care must be taken not to disturb the adjacent vagus nerves.

B. DIFFUSE ESOPHAGEAL SPASM

1. **General characteristics.** Diffuse esophageal spasm involves only the body of the esophagus, not the LES. It is less common than achalasia and is a benign condition that requires only symptomatic relief. Diffuse esophageal spasm occurs as a result of simultaneous, repetitive, or prolonged contractions that may have higher-than-normal amplitude.

Derby Hospitals NHS Foundation
Trust
Library and Knowledge Service

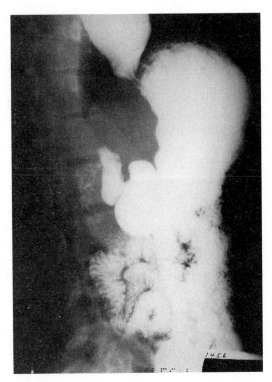

● **Figure 2.1** Barium swallow of a patient with achalasia. Note the "bird beak" appearance of the distal esophagus and the dilated proximal segment.

2. **Clinical features**
   a. Diffuse esophageal spasm causes more severe chest pain than achalasia. It may be confused with angina.
   b. Diffuse esophageal spasm causes less dysphagia than achalasia.
3. **Diagnosis**
   a. **Barium swallow** may show segmental spasm or esophageal diverticulum, which develops after prolonged disease.
   b. **Manometric studies** show repetitive, simultaneous esophageal contractions. These contractions may be prolonged. In contrast to achalasia, the esophagus maintains peristaltic ability.
4. **Treatment**
   a. **Medication.** Calcium channel blockers and long-acting nitrates often abolish symptoms.
   b. **Esophageal myotomy** is reserved for patients who have severe symptoms that are refractory to medical therapy. If myotomy is performed, the LES must also be divided because loss of esophageal peristalsis after myotomy prevents the propulsion of food past a competent LES. Therefore, a partial fundoplication must also be performed after the LES myotomy.

II Esophageal Diverticula and Webs

A. **ESOPHAGEAL DIVERTICULA**
   1. **General characteristics**
      a. Most esophageal diverticula are not congenital but develop during adulthood.

b. Esophageal diverticula are usually false diverticula. They are caused by herniation of mucosa and submucosa through the esophageal musculature. An example is **pharyngoesophageal (Zenker) diverticulum.**

c. Traction diverticula are true diverticula (i.e., evagination of all layers of the esophagus). They are caused by an inflammatory reaction in the mediastinal lymph nodes. This reaction produces a traction force on the esophagus that creates the diverticulum. These diverticula are relatively rare.

2. Clinical features of Zenker diverticulum

a. Zenker diverticulum occurs in people who are 30–50 years of age.

b. It arises within the inferior pharyngeal constrictor muscle above the cricopharyngeus muscle.

c. Symptoms may include cervical dysphagia, effortless regurgitation, a gurgling sensation in the neck on swallowing, and periodic aspiration.

3. Diagnosis is made with a barium esophagram, which shows the diverticulum.

4. Treatment. Surgical therapy is successful and involves a **cricopharyngeal myotomy.** This procedure relieves the relative obstruction distal to the diverticulum. The diverticulum itself may be left intact if it is smaller than 3 cm. Larger diverticula may be stapled off and excised.

B. ESOPHAGEAL WEB (SCHATZKI RING)

1. General characteristics. An esophageal web is an annular constriction of the distal esophagus. It is associated with a sliding hiatal hernia. The ring occurs at the squamocolumnar junction between the stomach and the esophagus.

2. Clinical features

a. Dysphagia is common and tends to occur when the diameter of the ring is approximately 15–20 mm.

b. Reflux symptoms (e.g., epigastric burning when lying flat that is relieved by meals and antacids) also may occur.

3. Diagnosis

a. **Barium esophagram** delineates the narrowing but does not differentiate it from esophagitis that causes a stricture.

b. **Esophagoscopy** is necessary to evaluate the mucosa and identify changes that indicate esophagitis leading to a stricture. This procedure is also used to identify tumors that might be mistaken for a web on a swallow study.

4. Treatment

a. Patients who have dysphagia tend to respond well only to periodic esophageal dilation with endoscopy.

b. Patients who also have reflux symptoms should undergo dilation and receive antireflux medical therapy (e.g., ranitidine).

c. Patients whose symptoms are refractory to this treatment should undergo operative dilation and an antireflux operation (Nissen fundoplication) to alleviate the hiatal hernia.

III Hiatal Hernia

A. GENERAL CHARACTERISTICS. There are two main types, I and II.

1. In **type I** hiatal hernia, the proximal stomach and intra-abdominal esophagus slide through the hiatus and into the mediastinum.

2. In **type II** hiatal hernia, the esophagus remains in its anatomic position, but the stomach slides adjacent to the esophagus through the hiatus (Figure 2-2).

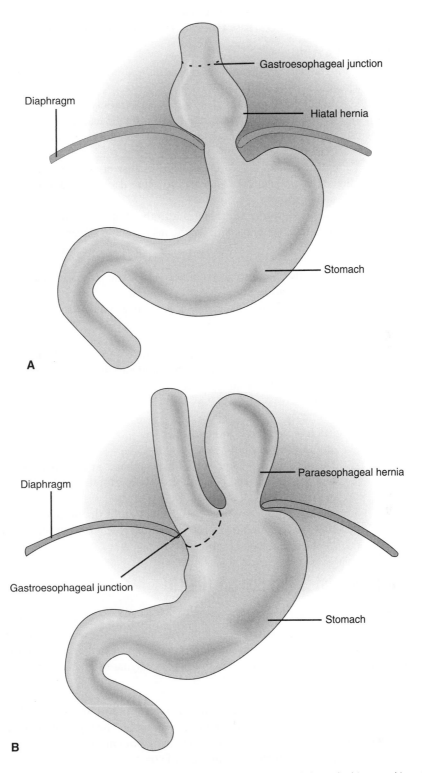

● **Figure 2.2** (*A*) Type I hiatal hernia. The gastroesophageal junction is displaced above the hiatus and into the thoracic cavity. (*B*) Type II hiatal hernia. The gastroesophageal junction is at its appropriate location; however, there is a para-esophageal herniation of the stomach.

3. **Type III** is a combination of types I and II. **Type IV** involves organs other than the stomach (e.g., colon). These types are less common than types I and II.

B. **CLINICAL FEATURES**
1. **Type I** hiatal hernia is usually an incidental radiographic finding. In some cases, it causes symptoms of reflux.
2. **Type II** hiatal hernia causes dysphagia, early satiety, a sensation of gurgling or splashing in the chest, and postprandial vomiting. Because the anatomic location of the esophagogastric junction tends to remain unaltered, reflux symptoms are not typically present.
   a. Patients may have a perforated ulcer because of poor gastric emptying of acid. Hemorrhagic ulcer may also lead to acute decompensation with hypotension and tachycardia.
   b. If most of the stomach herniates into the thoracic cavity, there is a significant risk of gastric volvulus with gastric necrosis and sepsis.

C. **DIAGNOSIS**
1. **Barium swallow** provides a dynamic view of the gastroesophageal junction and facilitates identification of the distorted anatomy.
2. **Esophagoscopy** allows visualization of reflux esophagitis.

D. **TREATMENT**
1. **Medical therapy** includes antacids [e.g., histamine (H_2) blockers, omeprazole]; avoidance of coffee, tobacco, and alcohol; and elimination of tight garments, which raise intra-abdominal pressure and increase reflux symptoms. Most patients respond to this management.
2. **Surgical therapy**
   a. Surgical intervention is indicated if:
      i. Medical therapy fails
      ii. The patient has a large type II hernia that is at increased risk for volvulus
      iii. The patient has acute symptoms of a perforated or hemorrhagic ulcer or gastric volvulus
   b. Surgical correction involves both reduction of the hernia and Nissen fundoplication with tightening of the crural defect to prevent reflux symptoms and recurrence of the hiatal hernia.

IV Gastroesophageal Reflux Disease (GERD)

A. **GENERAL CHARACTERISTICS.** GERD is usually caused by a defective LES. It is also associated with hiatal hernia and esophageal motility disorders. The condition may progress to esophagitis and can develop into Barrett's esophagus (columnar epithelialization of the distal esophagus), which is a premalignant state.

B. **CLINICAL FEATURES**
1. Patients typically have **heartburn and regurgitation** approximately 1 hour after meals. Lying flat may exacerbate these symptoms. The regurgitant has a bitter taste.
2. **Aspiration** may occur and lead to recurring **pneumonia.**
3. **Dysphagia** suggests the development of stricture or tumor.

C. **DIAGNOSIS**
1. **Barium swallow** may show an anatomic cause (e.g., hiatal hernia). However, findings may be normal.

2. **Esophagoscopy** may show esophagitis, stricture, or Barrett's esophagus. These are complications of GERD.
3. If these tests do not disclose the cause of the symptoms, **esophageal manometry** and **esophageal pH monitoring** will show prolonged relaxation of the LES in association with prolonged exposure of the lower esophagus to low pH. Esophageal motility disorders must be ruled out as the cause of symptoms because treatments differ.

D. TREATMENT
1. **Nonoperative.** Antacids (e.g., ranitidine) provide symptomatic relief. Omeprazole often provides superior relief in patients whose symptoms are refractory to H_2 blockers. If symptoms persist after 4 weeks of medical therapy, endoscopy should be performed to look for stricture, esophagitis, Barrett's esophagus, or tumor.
2. **Surgical.** Laparoscopic Nissen fundoplication is the most common surgical procedure. It involves performing a snug crural closure and wrapping the gastric fundus around the distal esophagus, which decreases reflux. Prerequisites for antireflux surgery include:
   a. Demonstration of GERD on 24-hour esophageal pH monitoring
   b. Symptoms or complications that occur despite adequate medical therapy
   c. GERD whose cause is amenable to surgical therapy (usually a defective LES)

V Esophageal Caustic Injury

A. GENERAL CHARACTERISTICS
1. Usually caused by accidental swallowing of household acid or alkali agents (e.g., bleach, detergents) in children as opposed to adults who intentionally ingest these agents as a suicide attempt.
2. Alkali agents produce more devastating liquefaction necrosis compared to acidic agents, which produce a coagulation necrosis that tends to limit the depth of injury.
3. Injury may be mild and require no specific therapy. Moderate injury often leads to strictures, while severe injuries produce perforation.

B. CLINICAL FEATURES
1. Upper airway injury may lead to stridor and hoarseness.
2. Esophageal injury presents with retrosternal pain and dysphagia.
3. Aspiration pneumonitis may result in hypoxia and shortness of breath.
4. If esophageal perforation develops, severe retrosternal chest pain, hypotension, fever, and sepsis ensue.
5. If perforation is present in the distal esophagus or stomach, the patient may complain of abdominal pain and have signs of peritonitis.

C. DIAGNOSIS
1. If esophageal perforation is suspected based on severity of symptoms, a contrast esophagram with gastrografin or dilute barium should be performed to assess for a leak.
2. Esophagoscopy should be performed in those who do not require immediate operation for perforation to assess the depth of the burn.
3. Chest radiograph may show mediastinum if perforation has occurred in the thoracic esophagus, while free intraperitoneal air may be present on abdominal series if distal esophageal or gastric perforation is present.

D. TREATMENT
1. Vomiting should **not** be induced as this increases esophageal exposure to the agent.

2. Patients with significant laryngeal edema and airway compromise should be intubated before the airway is lost.
3. Intravenous fluids should be administered to stabilize patients with hypovolemia.
4. Broad-spectrum antibiotics should be administered only if severe second- or third-degree burns are present to minimize bacteremia from translocation.
5. Those with severe burns must be monitored and kept NPO for several days to ensure that perforation does not develop.
6. Patients with perforation require immediate operation. An abdominal approach is favored to assess the stomach and distal esophagus. All necrotic esophagus must be removed and can be done through a transhiatal approach, thereby avoiding thoracotomy. The normal esophagus can be brought out of a cervical incision, and an esophageal cutaneous fistula (spit fistula) can be created. Restoration of intestinal continuity should not be restored during the initial operation because of the potential for significant edema and injury.
7. If a significant delay in the diagnosis occurs and extensive mediastinitis exists, a thoracic approach is necessary to appropriately clear out the infection and remove the damaged esophagus.
8. Patients with moderate injuries commonly develop strictures and can usually be managed with endoscopic balloon dilation. This procedure should not be performed until 6 weeks after the injury to allow reepithelialization of the esophagus, which reduces the risk of perforation from the procedure. Esophagectomy and colonic interposition for strictures is required if iatrogenic perforation occurs or if strictures are refractory to balloon dilation for 6–12 months. The stomach may be used instead of the colon; however, it often has associated damage and may not be ideal for an anastomosis.

VI Esophageal Neoplasms

A. GENERAL CHARACTERISTICS
1. Most esophageal tumors are malignant because the esophagus has no serosal layer. As a result, invasion into adjacent structures is common.
2. Malignant esophageal tumors include squamous cell carcinoma and adenocarcinoma.
3. The most common benign tumor is a leiomyoma.

B. LEIOMYOMA
1. **General characteristics**
   a. Leiomyomas occur in people 20–50 years of age.
   b. These tumors are usually located in the middle and lower segments rather than in the cervical esophagus.
   c. Tumors smaller than 5 cm rarely cause symptoms.
2. **Clinical features** include:
   a. Dysphagia
   b. Retrosternal pressure and pain
   c. Weight loss (if the discomfort associated with eating has resulted in decreased caloric intake)
   d. Obstruction and regurgitation (if the tumor encircles the esophagus)
   e. Malignant degeneration (rare)
3. **Diagnosis**
   a. **Barium esophagram** shows a concave submucosal defect with characteristic sharp borders and a smooth surface (Figure 2-3).

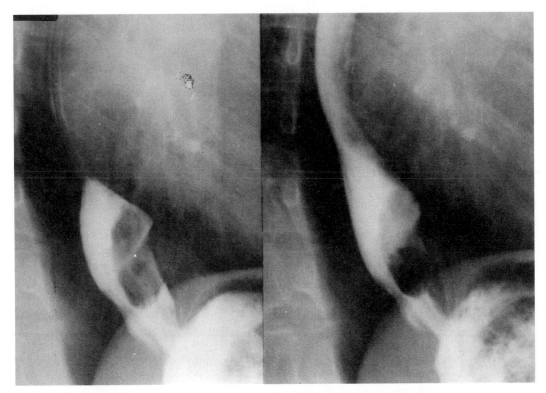

● **Figure 2.3** Barium swallow of a patient with leiomyoma of the esophagus. Note the smooth contour of the mucosa, suggesting a mural tumor rather than one that infiltrates the mucosa.

    b.   **Esophagoscopy** is required to visualize the mass. If the mucosa is intact and the findings on barium swallow suggest leiomyoma, an endoscopic biopsy should not be performed because the resultant mucosal scar may make extramural resection of the mass difficult.

    c.   **Endoscopic ultrasound** is a new modality that identifies leiomyoma as a distinct intramural mass of characteristic low density.

  4. **Treatment**

    a.   Asymptomatic or incidentally found leiomyoma can be safely followed with repeat barium swallow.

    b.   Masses larger than 5 cm and those that are symptomatic should be excised. Once resected, these tumors virtually never recur.

C. **SQUAMOUS CELL CARCINOMA**

  1. **General characteristics**

    a.   Worldwide, squamous cell carcinoma is the most common malignant tumor of the esophagus.

    b.   It most commonly occurs in elderly men.

    c.   The risk of squamous cell carcinoma is increased with cigarette smoking and alcohol consumption.

    d.   Tumors begin as multifocal areas of dysplasia (carcinoma in situ). The dysplasia progresses, invades the basement membrane, and gives rise to invasive squamous cell carcinoma. Advanced squamous cell carcinoma occurs when the tumor involves the muscle layers and beyond (Table 2-1).

TABLE 2-1	DISTRIBUTION OF SQUAMOUS CELL CARCINOMA OF THE ESOPHAGUS
Segment	**Percentage of Squamous Cell Tumors**
Cervical	8
Upper and midthoracic	55
Lower	37

    2. Clinical features include:

      a. Dysphagia

      b. GERD (if the tumor is associated with the LES)

      c. Weight loss and constitutional symptoms (e.g., malaise, low-grade fever, fatigue) with anorexia

      d. Metastatic disease (detectable by palpation of the supraclavicular lymph nodes)

    3. Diagnosis

      a. **Esophagoscopy** is required for identification and biopsy of the lesion. Esophagoscopy is used for the initial assessment because it is more sensitive than barium swallow.

      b. **Barium swallow** often shows an irregular filling defect.

      c. **Chest radiography** may show pulmonary hilar adenopathy or a pulmonary nodule.

      d. **Abdominal and chest computed tomography** scans are required to assess the patient for the presence of metastatic disease in the liver, the lung, and the celiac and tracheobronchial nodes.

        i. Metastatic disease is present in 75% of patients at diagnosis and is associated with a 5-year survival rate of 3%.

        ii. When no evidence of metastatic disease exists, the 5-year survival rate approaches 40%.

    4. Treatment

      a. If no metastatic disease is present, surgery offers the best chance at cure when esophageal resection and gastric pull-up and esophagogastric anastomosis are performed. If a considerable portion of the stomach must be resected to obtain clear margins, or if tension-free anastomosis of the stomach cannot be achieved, colonic interposition may be used.

      b. Neoadjuvant (treatment before surgery) radiation therapy and chemotherapy are useful in shrinking the tumor mass to facilitate surgical excision. Chemoradiation therapy has little effect on cure rates.

      c. Surgery may be offered to patients with metastatic disease for palliation. Patients who have significant obstructive symptoms may undergo a palliative resection with esophagogastric anastomosis. If life expectancy is poor or if the patient is a poor operative candidate, a proximal esophagostomy to the skin at the neck can be created with an ostomy bag for secretions. A gastrostomy tube can be placed to allow enteral feeding.

      d. Follow-up for patients who have lesions that are resected for cure includes esophagoscopy to rule out recurrence at 3-, 6-, and 12-month intervals. Recurring tumors tend to arise at the suture line.

D. ADENOCARCINOMA

    1. General characteristics

      a. Adenocarcinoma accounts for 5%–10% of primary esophageal cancers. Its incidence is on the rise in the United States because of the increased incidence of Barrett's esophagus.

    b.   The peak incidence is in the sixth decade of life. It is more common in men.

    c.   Adenocarcinoma usually involves the distal third of the esophagus.

    d.   Transmural invasion and lymphatic spread are usually present at diagnosis. The splenic hilar, celiac axis, and paraesophageal nodes are most commonly involved. The liver and lungs are common sites of metastases.

2. **Clinical features** include:

    a.   Severe GERD, which is strongly associated with the development of Barrett's esophagus

    b.   Weight loss and constitutional symptoms

    c.   Dysphagia

3. **Diagnosis**

    a.   **Barium swallow** shows a filling defect in the distal esophagus.

    b.   **Esophagoscopy** should be performed in patients who have severe GERD that is refractory to medical therapy for surveillance for the development of Barrett's esophagus. This procedure permits biopsy of suspicious lesions.

    c.   **Chest radiograph** may show metastatic disease.

4. **Treatment** is similar to that of squamous cell carcinoma. The 5-year survival rate is less than 10%.

Chapter 3

Disorders of the Stomach and Duodenum

I Peptic Ulcer Disease

A. GENERAL CHARACTERISTICS. Peptic ulcer disease involves ulceration of the stomach, the duodenum, or both. Risk factors include cigarette smoking, use of nonsteroidal anti-inflammatory drugs (NSAIDs), and infection with *Helicobacter pylori*.

B. DUODENAL ULCER
1. **General characteristics.** Duodenal ulcer is associated with decreased basal bicarbonate secretion in the proximal duodenum. The formation of duodenal ulcers depends on increased basal gastric acid secretion and increased gastric acid secretion in response to a meal. Basal gastrin levels are normal in untreated patients who have duodenal ulcer disease (unless the condition is secondary to Zollinger-Ellison syndrome).
2. **Clinical features**
   a. Duodenal ulcer is characterized by burning, stabbing, or gnawing epigastric pain. This pain is not usually referred and there are often few physical findings unless perforation has occurred.
   b. Ingestion of food or antacids often relieve pain.
   c. If perforation is present, patients have significant guarding and percussion tenderness. They may even present in shock with hypotension, tachycardia, and fever. Referred pain to the right shoulder may be present as a result of diaphragmatic irritation.
3. **Diagnosis**
   a. **Endoscopy** is the preferred method of diagnosis. This method allows for biopsy of suspicious lesions, and it is more sensitive and specific than barium radiography.
      i. Duodenal ulcers typically occur in the first and second portions of the duodenum.
      ii. Ulcers that occur in the third or fourth portion suggest an underlying gastrinoma.
   b. In the acute setting, when perforation is suspected, a **gastrografin swallow** is preferred over a barium swallow because it does not cause chemical peritonitis.
4. **Treatment**
   a. Nonoperative
      i. **Histamine (H$_2$) receptor antagonists** (e.g., cimetidine, ranitidine) bind to histamine receptors on parietal cells and inhibit acid secretion.
         (a) By 4 weeks, 70% of patients have healed ulcers.
         (b) The relapse rate is 15% while the patient receives maintenance therapy.
         (c) Ulcers recur in more than 50% of patients within 1 year if therapy is discontinued.
      ii. **Proton pump inhibitors** (e.g., omeprazole) block acid secretion.

    (a) By 2 weeks, 80% of patients have healed ulcers; 95% are healed by 4 weeks.

    (b) Compared with H_2 blockers, omeprazole provides superior ulcer healing and pain relief.

  iii. **Sucralfate** coats the ulcer base and mucosal surface. In this way, it allows ulcer healing while buffering the acidic environment. Healing rates are comparable to those of H_2 blockers, but sucralfate must be taken four times a day.

  iv. **Misoprostol** (prostaglandin analog) acts as an antisecretory agent. It yields healing results similar to those of H_2 blockers. Its main side effect is diarrhea, which is common.

  v. *Helicobacter pylori* **therapy** greatly reduces recurrence rates in patients who have *H. pylori*–associated ulcers. Triple therapy (i.e., metronidazole, bismuth, and amoxicillin) is most successful.

b. **Surgical intervention** is reserved for patients who have **hemorrhage, perforation,** or **obstruction** and for those whose symptoms are **intractable.**

  i. **Surgical options**

    (a) **Truncal vagotomy and pyloroplasty** involves transection of the truncal vagus nerves above the esophagogastric junction. This procedure reduces gastric acid secretion by approximately 70%. The ulcer recurrence rate is approximately 10%–15%. A pyloroplasty is performed because denervation of the stomach may cause impaired gastric emptying of solids (Figure 3-1).

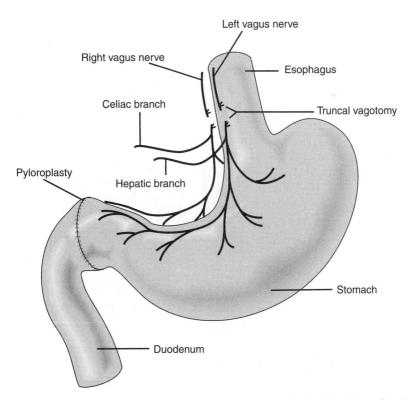

● **Figure 3.1** Truncal vagotomy and pyloroplasty. The vagus nerves are cut proximal to the division of any branches in the abdomen. Pyloroplasty is performed by making a longitudinal incision through the pylorus. The pylorus is sewn transversely to prevent narrowing.

(b) **Highly selective vagotomy** involves transecting the individual gastric fibers that supply the fundus but preserving the antropyloric fibers and the celiac and hepatic branches. This operation also reduces gastric acid secretion by approximately 70%. The ulcer recurrence rate is approximately 10%. However, highly selective vagotomy is more time-consuming than truncal vagotomy and pyloroplasty. Therefore, it may not be warranted in a critically ill patient (Figure 3-2).

(c) **Truncal vagotomy and antrectomy** involves transection of the truncal vagus nerves and removal of the antrum (Figure 3-3). It is accompanied by gastroduodenostomy (Billroth I procedure) or gastrojejunostomy (Billroth II procedure) to restore intestinal continuity (Figure 3-4). The antrectomy removes gastrin-secreting cells and further reduces gastric acid secretion (85%). It may also incorporate removal of the ulcer. The ulcer recurrence rate is very low (1%–2%).

ii. **Hemorrhage**

(a) Patients who have a history of previous hemorrhage have an increased risk of rebleed associated with their ulcer.

(b) Endoscopy identifies the bleeding site in 90% of patients. Attempts at endoscopic coagulation of the bleeding site are often successful.

(c) Patients should undergo surgical repair of the bleeding site if any of the following occur:

(i) Massive hemorrhage with shock

(ii) Prolonged blood loss that requires continued transfusions (usually >6 units)

(iii) Rebleeding after endoscopic therapy

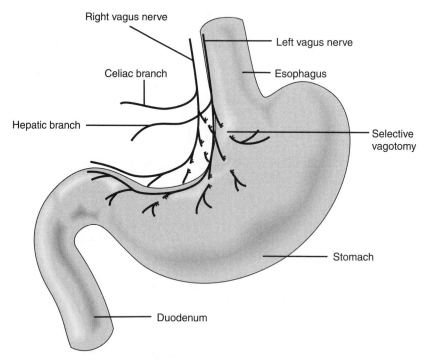

● Figure 3.2 Highly selective vagotomy. The specific branches of the vagus nerves, which innervate the stomach, are transected, leaving behind innervation to the pylorus to facilitate emptying.

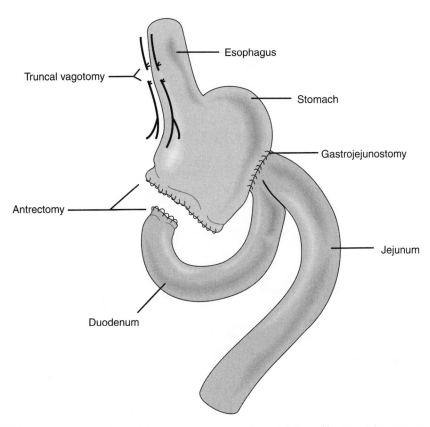

● **Figure 3.3** Vagotomy and antrectomy. A truncal vagotomy is performed, followed by gastrojejunostomy and resection of the antrum.

    (d) Acid reduction surgery (truncal vagotomy and pyloroplasty or truncal vagotomy and antrectomy) should be undertaken once the hemorrhage is controlled.

iii. **Perforation**

    (a) Patients who have evidence of perforation usually require surgical repair of the perforation with an omental patch (Figure 3-5).

    (b) As many as 70% of patients with acute perforation have recurrent ulcer disease if an antiulcer operation is not performed. Therefore, if the patient is stable at perforation repair, proximal gastric vagotomy with pyloroplasty, highly selective vagotomy or vagotomy and antrectomy should be strongly considered.

iv. **Obstruction**

    (a) Gastric outlet obstruction occurs acutely as a result of edematous inflammation at proximal duodenal ulcers. Chronic gastric outlet obstruction occurs when recurrent ulceration and scarring of the proximal duodenum cause a fixed stenosis.

    (b) Acute obstruction is treated conservatively with intravenous fluid, nasogastric tube decompression, and antisecretory agents. Obstruction usually resolves within 3–4 days.

    (c) Patients who have chronic obstruction must undergo upper endoscopy to exclude neoplasm as the cause. Balloon dilation can be used to relieve symptoms in most patients at endoscopy. However, recurrence is common, so surgical intervention is often necessary. Truncal vagotomy with

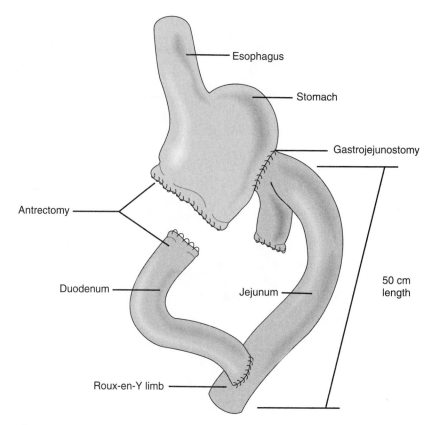

● **Figure 3.4** Billroth II procedure with Roux-en-Y reconstruction. The vagotomy, antrectomy, and gastrojejunostomy are performed as in Figure 3-3, but the proximal jejunum is diverted to a segment of bowel 50 cm distal to the gastrojejunostomy. This approach prevents bile reflux into the stomach and reduces the risk of alkaline gastritis.

antrectomy or pyloroplasty is often used to repair the obstruction and prevent recurrence.

    v. **Intractability**

        (a) Ulcers are defined as intractable if ulceration persists despite active medical therapy after 3 months or if they recur within 1 year despite maintenance therapy.

        (b) In this situation, surgery is not usually emergent. Therefore, the safest operation that provides adequate results and causes the least postoperative complications should be performed. Typically, this procedure is a highly selective vagotomy (Table 3-1).

5. Complications of ulcer surgery

    a. **Dumping syndrome** is caused by rapid entry of a food bolus into the proximal small bowel after pyloroplasty or antrectomy. There are two types, and they are characterized by their time of onset in relation to a meal.

        i. **Early dumping syndrome** typically occurs within 30 minutes of a meal. Patients may have epigastric pain, borborygmus, palpitations, dizziness, or syncope.

        (a) Meals that are high in carbohydrates (hyperosmolar) tend to cause more severe symptoms. High-carbohydrate meals are associated with a large inflow of extracellular fluid from the proximal bowel. This inflow is believed to cause the symptoms.

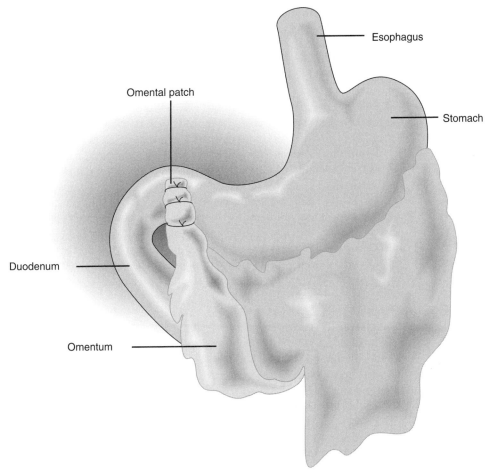

● **Figure 3.5** Omental patch for closure of a perforated gastroduodenal ulcer. Sutures are placed in the edges adjacent to the ulcer and then tied around a tail of omentum to seal the ulcer and provide a vascular pedicle for healing.

        (b) Patients should eat small meals and avoid fluid intake during meals. Fluid intake speeds gastric emptying and worsens symptoms. Most patients respond to diet changes.

    ii. **Late dumping syndrome** usually occurs 1–3 hours after a meal. It includes the symptoms of early dumping syndrome but is predominated by symptoms of hypoglycemia (e.g., diaphoresis, tachycardia, palpitations, fatigue, faintness).

TABLE 3-1	COMPARISON OF SURGICAL PROCEDURES FOR DUODENAL ULCER		
	HSV (%)	**TV (%)**	**TVA (%)**
Mortality	0	1	1.5
Ulcer relapse	10	10–15	<2
Dumping syndrome	<5	10	10–15
Diarrhea	<5	25	20

HSV = highly selective vagotomy; *TV* = truncal vagotomy; *TVA* = truncal vagotomy and antrectomy.

(a) The rapid increase in osmolar and carbohydrate load in the proximal small bowel causes a rapid and transient increase in blood sugar level. As a result, a burst of insulin is released and leads to hypoglycemia.

(b) **Octreotide** is useful in patients whose symptoms persist despite dietary changes. It slows intestinal transit and reduces peak plasma insulin levels.

b. **Alkaline reflux gastritis** occurs when bile refluxes into the stomach after ulcer surgery (either vagotomy and pyloroplasty or vagotomy and antrectomy). The incidence of persistent symptoms is less than 2%.

 i. **Symptoms.** Patients have postprandial epigastric pain, nausea and vomiting, endoscopic visualization of bile in the stomach, and histologic evidence of gastritis.

 ii. **Diagnosis.** Endoscopy must be performed to obtain a diagnosis because this symptom complex is also seen with recurrent ulcer disease, which may occur after unsuccessful surgery or Zollinger-Ellison syndrome.

 iii. **Treatment.** Surgical intervention is the only proven therapy. Typically, a Roux-en-Y gastrojejunostomy with an intestinal limb of 50–60 cm is sufficient to divert the intestinal contents away from the stomach (see Figure 3-4).

C. GASTRIC ULCER

1. General characteristics

a. Gastric ulcers are less common than duodenal ulcers in the United States. They are more common in Japan and are usually seen in elderly men.

b. These ulcers are classified according to location. The importance of acid secretion rates and surgical therapy varies with ulcer location (Figure 3-6).

c. Associated factors include tobacco, NSAIDs, steroids, stress, and *H. pylori* infection.

d. Gastric ulcers must be differentiated from ulcers associated with gastric malignancy.

2. Clinical features

a. Patients may have gnawing, dull, or burning pain in the epigastrium or left upper quadrant.

b. Some patients have nausea, vomiting, anorexia, and weight loss.

c. Pain may be aggravated by food.

d. Acute ulceration may occur with hemorrhage (vomiting frank blood, or coffee-ground emesis with or without heme-positive or melanotic stool) or perforation (acute onset of severe abdominal pain with guarding and worsening shock).

3. Diagnosis

a. **Barium swallow** is less expensive than endoscopy. However, 5% of malignant gastric ulcers are misdiagnosed as benign on contrast radiography.

b. **Upper endoscopy** is the most reliable method of diagnosis. It also permits biopsy of the ulcer to rule out malignancy. Endoscopy is indicated in patients who have suspected gastric ulcer accompanied by significant weight loss or anemia.

c. In the acute setting, free air on an **upright chest radiograph** indicates perforation. Often, this is the only diagnostic test required before surgery.

4. Treatment

a. **Nonsurgical therapy** is similar to that for duodenal ulcers.

b. **Surgical treatment** depends on the ulcer type and the presence of complications (e.g., hemorrhage, obstruction, perforation).

 i. **Elective surgery.** Ulcers that do not heal after 12 weeks of medical therapy, recurrent ulcers that do not respond to medical therapy, and the inability to exclude malignant disease are indications for elective surgery.

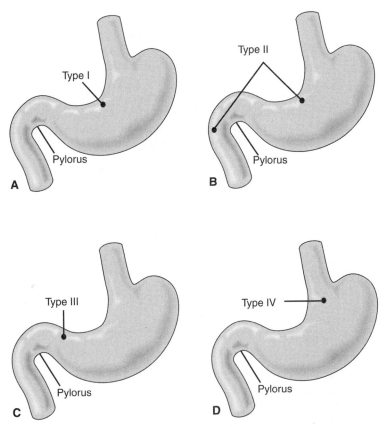

● **Figure 3.6** Ulcer location and acid secretion. (*A*) Type I ulcers are located on the lesser curvature of the stomach. They are not associated with increased acid secretion. (*B*) Type II ulcers are gastric and duodenal ulcers that are associated with increased acid secretion. (*C*) Type III ulcers are prepyloric ulcers that are associated with increased acid secretion. (*D*) Type IV ulcers are near the cardia and are not associated with increased acid secretion.

(a) **Type I.** These ulcers are not associated with hypersecretion of acid. Therefore, vagotomy is unnecessary and does not improve ulcer recurrence rates. However, vagotomy does increase rates of postvagotomy diarrhea. The procedure of choice is distal gastrectomy to include the ulcer with a Billroth I procedure. A Billroth II procedure should be used if the gastroduodenostomy is not technically feasible, but this approach is less physiologic.

(b) **Type II.** These ulcers are associated with hypersecretion of acid. Removal of the gastric antrum (incorporating the ulcer in the resection) reduces the risk of recurrence because this location is susceptible to these ulcers. Truncal vagotomy in conjunction with antrectomy further reduces the recurrence rate by further reducing acid secretion. A Billroth I reconstruction is recommended, but it may not be feasible if there is significant inflammation and scarring because of duodenal ulceration. In these cases, a Billroth II procedure is necessary.

(c) **Type III.** These ulcers are also associated with acid hypersecretion. They are treated similarly to type II ulcers.

(d) **Type IV.** Excision of the ulcer and distal gastrectomy with gastroduodenostomy is the procedure of choice. Vagotomy is not necessary because these patients do not hypersecrete acid.

ii. **Emergent surgery**
   (a) In patients who are critically unstable, surgery for **hemorrhage** should include ligation of the bleeding vessel and vagotomy with pyloroplasty. This procedure can be performed quickly and has the lowest mortality rate. In patients who are more stable, the acid reduction surgery should be done as outlined for elective procedures. Biopsy specimens should be taken to rule out malignancy.
   (b) Surgery for **perforation** in unstable patients involves biopsy of the ulcer and omental patch with vagotomy.
   (c) **Gastric outlet obstruction is not an emergency.** Patients who have gastric outlet obstruction should undergo decompression with a nasogastric tube, rehydration with intravenous fluids, and correction of electrolyte imbalances. Obstructing ulcers are usually type II or III. Therefore, these patients should undergo vagotomy with antrectomy and reconstruction with a Billroth I or II procedure.

Ⅱ Gastric Neoplasms

Common types of gastric neoplasms include adenocarcinoma, gastric lymphoma, and leiomyosarcoma.

A. ADENOCARCINOMA

1. **General characteristics**
   a. The **incidence** of malignant tumors is highest in Japan. It is likely diet related.
   b. The **risk of malignancy is increased** in patients who have gastric polyps (typically adenomatous polyps; hyperplastic polyps carry no malignant potential). Chronic gastritis and pernicious anemia are also associated with an increased risk of malignancy.
   c. The **5-year survival rates** for adenocarcinoma are dismal because the disease is often advanced at diagnosis (Tables 3-2 and 3-3).

2. **Clinical features**
   a. Patients have constant, nonradiating epigastric pain.
   b. Antacids may provide temporary relief.
   c. As the disease progresses, anorexia, nausea, and weight loss become apparent.
   d. Dysphagia may be present if lesions are located near the gastroesophageal junction.
   e. Perforation or acute hemorrhage is the presenting symptom in fewer than 10% of patients.
   f. Approximately 20% of patients have melena.
   g. Cachexia, hepatomegaly, and supraclavicular lymphadenopathy (Virchow's node) are indications of metastasis.

TABLE 3-2	FIVE-YEAR SURVIVAL RATES FOR GASTRIC ADENOCARCINOMA BY STAGE

Stage	Survival Rate (%)
I	90–95
II	40–50
III	10–15
IV	5–10

TABLE 3-3	TNM STAGING DEFINITIONS	
Stage	**TNM Classification**	**Definition**
I	T1, N0, M0	Tumor confined to mucosa; no nodes; no metastasis
II	T2–3, N0, M0	Tumor invading mucosa (T2); may penetrate serosa (T3); no nodes; no metastasis
III	T1–3, N1–2, M0	Tumor size as above; nodes in immediate vicinity of tumor (N1) or along gastric curvatures (N2); no metastasis
IV		Tumor unresectable or metastatic

3. **Diagnosis**
   a. **Upper endoscopy** with biopsy provides a definitive diagnosis in more than 95% of patients. It is the diagnostic method of choice.
   b. **Contrast radiography** is only 80%–90% accurate.
   c. **Computed tomography (CT) scans** often underestimate regional or distant lymph node involvement. Therefore, these scans are not a reliable staging tool. However, they are useful in detecting hepatic metastases.

4. **Treatment**
   a. **Surgical resection** offers the only chance for cure of **gastric adenocarcinoma.** Therefore, patients who have advanced disease at surgery should undergo palliative surgery to decrease symptoms and possibly eliminate obstruction.
      i. When curative resection is performed, margins of 5–6 cm around the tumor should be included. Surgical resection may be curative in patients who have lesions that do not penetrate the serosa and are not associated with lymph node spread.
      ii. Controversy exists over the benefit of radical celiac and peripancreatic nodal resection.
      iii. Palliative surgery for dysphagia or pain should be undertaken when endoscopic laser fulguration does not provide relief. Total gastric resection with esophagojejunostomy and Roux-en-Y anastomosis is often used for proximal lesions.
   b. **Chemoradiation therapy** offers little improvement in 5-year survival rates.

B. **GASTRIC LYMPHOMA**
   1. **General characteristics**
      a. The peak incidence occurs in the sixth and seventh decades.
      b. The histologic type is non-Hodgkin's lymphoma.
      c. In primary gastric lymphoma, the initial symptoms are gastric and the stomach is exclusively or predominantly involved. Otherwise, the diagnosis is systemic lymphoma with secondary gastric involvement.
   2. **Clinical features** include:
      a. Epigastric, nonradiating pain
      b. Weight loss and anorexia
      c. Nausea and vomiting
      d. Fecal occult blood and anemia (common)
      e. Gross hemorrhage (uncommon)
   3. **Diagnosis**
      a. **Endoscopy** is the diagnostic method of choice because biopsy and brush cytology provides the diagnosis in 90% of cases.

b. **Staging** should be done after endoscopic biopsy. Staging includes the following:
 i. CT scans of the chest and abdomen to identify other sites of lymphadenopathy
 ii. Bone marrow biopsy
 iii. Biopsy of enlarged palpable peripheral lymph nodes
 4. **Treatment**
 a. **Gastric resection** may be curative in patients whose tumor is confined to the stomach.
 b. **Radiation therapy** to the gastric bed is often used to reduce local recurrence.
 c. **Systemic chemotherapy** is needed when cancer spreads to the perigastric lymph nodes. These patients often have recurrence outside the radiation field.

C. LEIOMYOSARCOMA
 1. **General characteristics**
 a. Leiomyosarcoma is the most common sarcoma of the stomach.
 b. Leiomyosarcoma must be differentiated histologically from leiomyoma, which is benign.
 c. These tumors usually occur in the sixth and seventh decades.
 2. **Clinical features**
 a. Symptoms are identical to those of gastric adenocarcinoma.
 b. If the tumor is large, an epigastric mass may be palpable.
 3. **Diagnosis**
 a. **Endoscopy** is most often used to investigate patient symptoms. The tumor may be difficult to see endoscopically because it may not alter the overlying mucosa. However, a mass effect may be noted. When a submucosal mass is suspected, endoscopic ultrasound may be helpful in identifying its extent.
 b. **Contrast radiography** may help to delineate the mass.
 c. Histologically, tumors with **more than 5–10 mitoses** per 10 high-power fields have a higher metastatic rate.
 4. **Treatment**
 a. Chemotherapy does not increase survival.
 b. These tumors are not radiosensitive. Therefore, **surgical excision** is the treatment of choice. The tumor typically does not spread to the lymph nodes, so extensive lymphadenectomy is not indicated. En bloc resection of the tumor and involved structures should be attempted because negative surgical margins are necessary for cure.
 c. The 5-year survival rate for low-grade lesions is 80%. The 5-year survival rate for high-grade lesions is only 35%.

ⅠⅠⅠ Zollinger-Ellison Syndrome

A. GENERAL CHARACTERISTICS
 1. The tumor associated with Zollinger-Ellison syndrome is a pancreatic endocrine neoplasm that secretes gastrin (i.e., gastrinoma). This tumor causes recurrent gastroduodenal ulcers as a result of gastrin-stimulated hypersecretion of acid.
 2. Most cases occur sporadically, but approximately 25% are associated with multiple endocrine neoplasia I (MEN I) syndrome.
 3. Zollinger-Ellison syndrome is suspected in patients who have recurrent ulcers after acid reduction surgery or failure of medical therapy.

B. CLINICAL FEATURES

1. Symptoms are similar to those of peptic ulcer disease.
2. More than 50% of patients have diarrhea in addition to symptoms of peptic ulcer disease.

C. DIAGNOSIS

1. **Endoscopy** to confirm the presence of gastroduodenal ulceration may also show prominent rugae. These are associated with increased gastrin stimulation. Esophagitis may also be present.
2. Venous levels of gastrin higher than 1000 pg/mL are diagnostic of gastrinoma. In the face of elevated basal gastric acid output, gastrin levels higher than 200 pg/mL are also indicative of gastrinoma. The normal negative feedback mechanisms of high acid output usually decrease gastrin levels to much lower levels.
3. Gastrinoma must be differentiated from antral G-cell hyperplasia or simple hyperfunction of antral G cells when gastrin levels are lower than 1000 pg/mL. The **secretin stimulation test** is performed in the fasting state, and serial gastrin levels are measured. Elevation of more than 200 pg/mL above basal gastrin levels indicates gastrinoma.
4. Once the diagnosis is established, an attempt at tumor localization and staging must be made. CT scan may identify the tumor location or may identify hepatic metastasis. It is often the first modality used. If hepatic metastasis is identified, tissue biopsy must be obtained for confirmation.

D. TREATMENT

1. After ulcer disease is identified and the diagnosis of gastrinoma is made, acid secretion is effectively blocked by **omeprazole.** In almost all patients, the ulcer heals.
2. The tumor has malignant potential. Therefore, if it is resectable, localization and resection should be attempted.
   a. Most tumors occur in the **gastrinoma triangle.** This area is bounded superiorly by the cystic duct, inferiorly by the third portion of the duodenum, and medially by the neck of the pancreas (Figure 3-7).
   b. The entire abdomen must be evaluated at surgery for extrapancreatic or extraduodenal tumor. If no tumor is found in the pancreas or surrounding tissue, a duodenotomy must be performed to search for intraluminal gastrinoma. If it is present, the lesions are locally excised and the defects repaired.
   c. Pancreatic lesions smaller than 2 cm can be enucleated without a formal pancreatic resection. Large tumors or tumors that are deeply situated in the pancreas require partial pancreatectomy. Distal pancreatectomy is performed for distal lesions. Pancreaticoduodenectomy is performed for proximal lesions.
3. Total gastrectomy is reserved for patients who are noncompliant with omeprazole therapy. This treatment does not rid the patient of the gastrinoma, but it eliminates the primary symptom.
4. Chemotherapy does not improve survival.

IV Ampullary Lesions

A. GENERAL CHARACTERISTICS

1. Tumors are located at or near the ampulla of Vater. The tumors may be malignant or benign. Regardless of their malignant potential, they cause symptoms as a result of pancreaticobiliary obstruction.

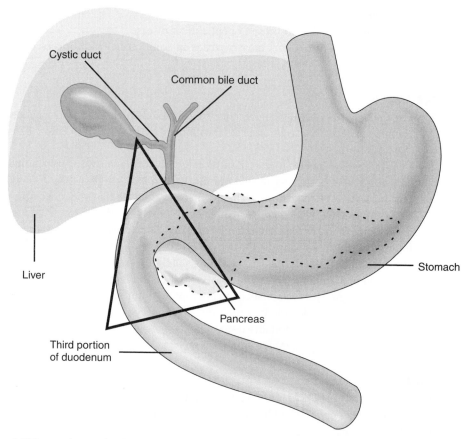

● **Figure 3.7** The gastrinoma triangle shows the boundaries within which most gastrinomas are found. These borders are formed by the cystic duct superiorly, the head of the pancreas medially, and the third portion of the duodenum inferiorly.

    2. Most of these tumors are adenocarcinoma of the head of the pancreas. Other possible sites of origin are the ampulla, distal common bile duct, and duodenum.

    3. Tumors tend to occur after the sixth decade. However, if they are associated with a familial polyposis syndrome, they can occur by the third decade.

B. CLINICAL FEATURES

    1. **Anorexia** and **weight loss** may be the initial symptoms.

    2. Epigastric abdominal **discomfort** and **nausea** may develop.

    3. **Pruritic jaundice** eventually develops when the tumor causes biliary obstruction. It may be associated with significant right upper quadrant pain that may progress to ascending cholangitis.

    4. **Pancreatitis** (severe epigastric pain with vomiting and hyperamylasemia) in an older patient who has no history of alcohol or gallstones must be investigated for periampullary tumor that causes pancreatic duct obstruction.

    5. **Profuse vomiting** because of duodenal obstruction may occur at a late stage.

    6. Transient melanotic stools or occult-positive stool with iron-deficiency anemia also may occur because these tumors can bleed intermittently.

C. DIAGNOSIS

    1. Biliary obstructive disease is indicated by elevated alkaline phosphatase and conjugated bilirubin levels with mildly elevated or normal transaminase levels.

2. An **elevated CA-19–9** level is 90% sensitive and specific for tumors that originate in the pancreas.

3. **Ultrasound** is often the first modality used to evaluate patients because the more common cause of biliary obstruction is gallstones. These are readily seen on ultrasound of the gallbladder.
   a. Dilated intrahepatic and extrahepatic ducts can also be identified. A dilated common bile duct is usually larger than 0.8–1.0 cm.
   b. If no gallstones are identified and biliary obstruction is seen, the ultrasound may identify an abnormality in the head of the pancreas. However, intraluminal tumors at the ampulla are usually difficult to see because of the presence of duodenal gas.

4. **CT scan** is useful in patients who have biliary or pancreatic duct obstruction when gallstones have been ruled out. CT scan can identify pancreatic masses as small as 2 cm and can detect metastases. It may even detect an ampullary mass.

5. **Endoscopic retrograde cholangiopancreatography (ERCP)** is necessary for patients with biliary obstruction.
   a. It provides a means to diagnose an ampullary tumor if CT scan does not identify a pancreatic mass.
   b. It allows placement of a stent to relieve the biliary obstruction until definitive surgery is performed.

6. **Endoscopic biopsy** of periampullary lesions has a considerable false-negative rate (sometimes as high as 30%–40%). Therefore, the finding of an adenoma (benign) as opposed to an adenocarcinoma (malignant) on an endoscopic biopsy specimen should not give the surgeon or the patient a false sense of security.

D. TREATMENT

1. Surgical therapy for **pancreatic lesions** is the same as for pancreatic cancer.

2. **Periampullary lesions** may be adenocarcinoma of the duodenum or a benign adenoma, as determined by endoscopic biopsy. All of these lesions require resection to provide a definitive diagnosis, relieve obstructive symptoms, and remove a possible malignancy.
   a. Patients who are medically fit should be offered pancreaticoduodenectomy to remove the lesion, even if initial biopsy specimens show benign adenoma (because of the significant false-negative rate). This approach offers the best chance for cure (5-year survival rate of 40%).
   b. Patients who are not medically fit should undergo local resection of the tumor mass with pancreatic and biliary duct reanastomosis to the duodenum. This approach provides effective palliation of symptoms and carries an overall 5-year survival rate of 25%–30%.
   c. Patients who refuse surgery can obtain symptomatic relief with biliary stenting.

Chapter 4

Disorders of the Small Intestine

I. Small Bowel Obstruction

A. GENERAL CHARACTERISTICS. Small bowel obstruction is usually caused by adhesions formed after previous abdominal surgery or from bowel located within an incarcerated hernia. Other causes include obstruction by neoplasms (primary small bowel neoplasms or metastases), volvulus (twisting of the bowel), strictures associated with Crohn's disease, infection with an obstructing abscess, and intussusception. Small bowel obstruction can occur at any age. It must be differentiated from ileus, which is managed nonoperatively.

B. CLINICAL FEATURES. The presentation varies depending on the cause.
1. Patients who have a hernia or adhesions usually have anorexia and crampy abdominal pain, usually in the low and middle abdomen. The pain may have a wavelike crescendo/decrescendo quality, with periods of minimal discomfort in between waves.
2. Eventually, nausea and vomiting occur.
3. Patients who have a complete obstruction may report the absence of bowel movements and flatus. Patients who have a partial obstruction may pass only small amounts of liquid stool or only flatus with no bowel movements.
4. Fever should alert the physician to the possibility of bowel compromise or perforation.
5. Examination typically shows generalized tenderness and a distended abdomen that is tympanic to percussion. There is minimal guarding or percussion tenderness if no bowel compromise has occurred. Careful inspection for previous scars and palpation of the scar sites for incisional hernia must be performed. The groin and umbilicus must also be assessed for a hernia.
6. If guarding is present or if the pain has progressed from intermittent cramps to continuous pain, bowel compromise may be present. These patients may have signs of sepsis, including tachycardia and hypotension.
7. Auscultation typically shows peristaltic rushes with high-pitched bowel sounds and tinkling. In contrast, in ileus, bowel sounds are nearly absent.
8. Rectal examination typically shows minimal stool in the rectum. This examination may also show occult blood, depending on the cause of the obstruction.

C. DIAGNOSIS
1. **Blood tests.** An elevated white blood cell count suggests compromised bowel. Anemia may signal a neoplastic process as the cause. Lactic acidosis may be present if significant bowel infarction or ischemia has occurred secondary to strangulation.
2. **An abdominal series** typically shows a stepladder pattern of air–fluid levels, with dilated small bowel proximal to the site of obstruction. Minimal gas and stool are typically seen in the colon and rectum (Figure 4-1).
3. In a patient who has no evidence of a hernia and no previous surgeries, the etiology of the small bowel obstruction is unclear. **Computed tomography (CT) scan** may

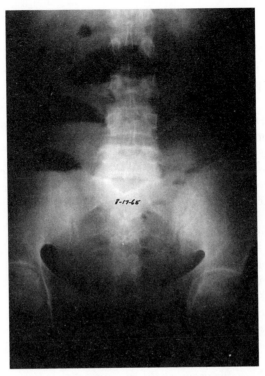

● **Figure 4.1** Abdominal series showing the classic appearance of a small bowel obstruction. There are multiple loops of distended small bowel with air–fluid levels. Minimal gas is seen in the colon and rectum.

help to identify a mass as the cause. The CT scan may identify metastatic disease, or it may show a volvulus with signs of bowel compromise. In the case of bowel compromise, early operation is needed to prevent septic complications associated with bowel death and perforation.

4. If the distinction between ileus and bowel obstruction is difficult, a **barium small bowel series** can be used to identify an obstruction. If an ileus is present, the contrast material will take an extended period to reach the colon (usually >4 hours), but no obstruction site will be seen.

D. TREATMENT

1. Patients who do not have signs of bowel compromise should undergo nasogastric decompression to relieve their symptoms. These patients also require aggressive intravenous fluid rehydration and serial examinations to detect compromised bowel. If the obstruction appears to be complete, is believed to be caused by adhesions, and does not resolve after a short course of observation (12 hours) with the above measures, surgery is indicated to lyse the adhesions.

2. Patients who have bowel compromise with peritoneal signs should undergo immediate operation.

3. If a hernia is present, an attempt should be made to reduce it. If the hernia is not reducible and an obstruction is present, the hernia is incarcerated. In this case, surgery is needed to repair the hernia and relieve the obstruction.

4. If peritoneal signs are present and the hernia mass is extremely tender, perforation or strangulation of the bowel may be present. In this case, surgery must be undertaken emergently to repair the hernia. If the bowel segment does not appear viable, it must be resected.

5. If the hernia is reducible with pressure, the patient should be observed for 12–24 hours or given specific instructions to watch for signs of worsening abdominal pain and fever. The patient should undergo elective hernia repair to prevent recurrence.

Ⅱ Small Bowel Neoplasms

A. GENERAL CHARACTERISTICS. Primary neoplasms of the small bowel are rare. Benign tumors are more common.

1. The most common **benign** tumors are leiomyomas and adenomas. These tumors are usually asymptomatic unless they become large and cause obstruction.

2. Adenocarcinoma is the most common **malignant** neoplasm, followed closely by carcinoid. Leiomyosarcoma and lymphoma are less common malignancies.

B. ADENOMA is classified as tubular or villous.

1. **Tubular adenomas** have a low malignant potential. They may be amenable to endoscopic polypectomy because they are often pedunculated. If this procedure is not easily accomplished because of the location of the adenoma (i.e., out of endoscopic reach, past the duodenum) or because the adenoma is not pedunculated, then surgical excision is performed to relieve symptoms and avoid the small risk of malignancy.

2. **Villous adenomas** have malignant potential and require excision. They are often seen in the familial polyposis syndromes and often occur in the periampullary region.

C. LEIOMYOMA usually occurs in the jejunum.

1. **Diagnosis.** Contrast radiography may show a filling defect with a smooth surface. A palpable mass may be present if the tumor is large.

2. **Sequelae.** Eventually, these tumors outgrow their blood supply and may ulcerate, producing intraluminal bleeding. Occasionally, they cause obstructive symptoms, but this outcome is less common because their growth tends to be extraluminal rather than intraluminal.

3. **Treatment** requires surgical resection to alleviate symptoms and to differentiate these tumors from their malignant counterpart, leiomyosarcoma.

D. ADENOCARCINOMA

1. **General characteristics.** Adenocarcinoma is the most common malignant tumor of the small intestine. It arises from the epithelial cells of the small intestinal mucosa. Adenocarcinoma tends to occur in the sixth and seventh decades. In younger patients, it may be associated with Crohn's disease.

2. **Clinical features**
   a. Weight loss
   b. Crampy abdominal pain caused by intermittent bouts of obstruction
   c. Symptoms related to pancreaticobiliary obstruction
   d. Occult blood in stool
   e. Palpable mass (usually not present because these tumors grow intraluminally) or small bowel obstruction

3. **Diagnosis**
   a. **Blood tests** may show anemia.
   b. A **plain abdominal series** may show evidence of small bowel obstruction.
   c. **Endoscopy** is useful for periampullary lesions. Lesions that are past the duodenum are typically out of reach of conventional upper endoscopy.
   d. **Contrast radiography** may show a filling defect with ulceration (Figure 4-2).
   e. **CT scan** may identify a mass that is larger than 2 cm.

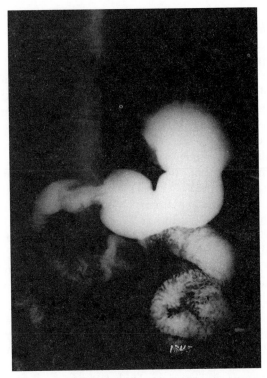

● **Figure 4.2** Barium small bowel follow-through shows a mass lesion in the small bowel. The mass has an irregular border, suggesting small bowel adenocarcinoma. The lesion is seen inferior to the antrum at the fourth portion of the duodenum.

    4. Treatment
       a. **Wide surgical resection** that includes the draining nodal system offers the best chance for cure.
          i. Tumors of the duodenum typically require pancreaticoduodenectomy to incorporate the draining nodes, which may contain cancer.
          ii. Palliative surgery for unresectable, obstructing duodenal lesions may be achieved by gastrojejunostomy.
          iii. Jejunoileal lesions are removed by segmental resection that includes the root of the mesentery (to include the draining nodes to the segment).
          iv. Distal ileal tumors are treated by right hemicolectomy that includes the ileal tumor because the nodal drainage includes the nodes associated with the right colon.
       b. Radiation therapy and chemotherapy are not beneficial.
       c. The overall 5-year survival rate is less than 30% and is related to the presence of nodal metastasis at diagnosis. In patients without nodal involvement, the survival rate may be as high as 60%–70% after resection.

E. CARCINOID
    1. General characteristics
       a. The frequency of carcinoid is similar to that of adenocarcinoma of the small bowel.
       b. The peak incidence is in the sixth decade.
       c. Approximately 20%–30% of patients have a synchronous noncarcinoid neoplasm. The neoplasm is usually found in the colon, lung, stomach, or breast.
       d. Carcinoid tumors originate from cells of the amine precursor uptake decarboxylase (APUD) system. The specific cell involved is the Kulchitsky cell, which is found in the crypts of Lieberkühn.

e. Most carcinoid tumors occur in the appendix. The small intestine is the next most common site of origin, although tumors can occur anywhere in the intestinal tract.

f. The carcinoid syndrome (see below) may develop.

2. **Clinical features**

a. Most tumors are small and asymptomatic and are found at autopsy.

b. Small bowel obstruction may occur in association with tumor growth and tethering of the small bowel mesentery. Kinking of the intestine also may occur.

c. Intestinal bleeding is unusual.

d. Anorexia, fatigue, and weight loss also may be present. These symptoms are usually a sign of metastatic disease.

e. **Carcinoid syndrome** typically occurs when there is a large bulk of tumor metastatic to the liver. These tumors secrete serotonin. Its release produces the following characteristic symptoms:

   i. Intermittent flushing and diarrhea are common.

   ii. Bronchospasm, venous telangiectasia of the face, and pellagra (i.e., dementia, diarrhea, and dermatitis) are less common.

   iii. Carcinoid crisis (i.e., tachyarrhythmias, profound hypertension or hypotension, generalized flushing, and severe diarrhea) is uncommon.

3. **Diagnosis**

a. **CT scan** is useful for identifying the primary tumor and for evaluating regional node and liver metastases.

b. **Endoscopy** typically is not useful because only a minority of carcinoid tumors are found in the proximal small bowel.

c. **Laboratory test.** The urinary level of 5-hydroxyindoleacetic acid (5-HIAA), which is a breakdown product of serotonin, is typically elevated in patients who have carcinoid syndrome.

d. Because carcinoid is associated with other malignancies, patients should undergo **colonoscopy** and **upper endoscopy** to rule out a synchronous lesion.

e. These tumors are slow growing. Therefore, the 5-year survival rate is approximately 60%. Once liver metastases are present, the median survival is 3 years.

4. **Treatment**

a. Wide en bloc excision that includes the nodal draining system should be performed. Therefore, tumors that involve the distal ileum should be resected with a **right hemicolectomy.** Appendiceal carcinoids that are smaller than 2 cm can be treated by appendectomy alone.

b. **Resection.** Isolated hepatic metastases should be considered for resection. However, liver metastases are usually multiple and are not amenable to resection.

c. **Inspection.** Because these tumors are multicentric, the entire bowel must be inspected for another primary carcinoid tumor. Further, the association with other noncarcinoid malignancies mandates a thorough intraoperative inspection.

d. **Radiation** therapy offers no benefit. Response rates for **chemotherapy** are only 20%–30%.

e. **Octreotide** is effective in treating the symptoms of carcinoid syndrome and carcinoid crisis. Octreotide decreases circulating serotonin levels and decreases symptoms.

F. **LEIOMYOSARCOMA**

1. **General characteristics**

a. Peak incidence is during the sixth decade. However, this type of tumor can occur at any age.

b. Leiomyosarcomas arise from the muscularis mucosa. They tend to occur in the jejunoileal region.

c. Leiomyosarcomas tend to arise in Meckel's diverticulum.

2. Clinical features

  a. These tumors grow extraluminally. As a result, symptoms of obstruction do not occur until the tumor is relatively large.

  b. Weight loss and abdominal pain are the most common presenting symptoms.

  c. Pain may be associated with hemorrhage caused by necrosis. The hemorrhage may be intraluminal. Therefore, gastrointestinal bleeding or occult blood may be detected on rectal examination. The tumor may bleed within itself or into the abdominal cavity, producing peritoneal signs.

  d. A mass is often palpable at presentation.

3. Diagnosis

  a. **Contrast radiography** may show a filling defect and mass effect.

  b. Because these tumors often cause a palpable mass, **CT scan** is the most useful tool for imaging the lesion. Metastatic disease to the liver or other parts of the abdomen may also be identified.

  c. Because these tumors are often found in the distal gastrointestinal tract, endoscopy is not usually helpful.

  d. Definitive diagnosis relies on **surgical excision.**

  e. Survival is best predicted by histologic grade. Low-grade tumors have a low number of mitotic figures. The 5-year survival rate for these tumors is 70%. The 5-year survival rate for high-grade tumors is less than 20%.

4. Treatment

  a. **Wide en bloc resection** with the associated mesentery is necessary for an attempt at cure. Chemoradiation therapy offers no benefit.

  b. Extended lymphadenectomy is not indicated because these tumors usually do not spread through the lymphatic system.

  c. Resection of isolated pulmonary or hepatic metastases may prolong survival. However, this effect has not been well studied.

G. LYMPHOMA

1. General characteristics

  a. Lymphoma may occur as primary lymphoma of the small bowel with associated peripheral lymphadenopathy or splenomegaly. It may also occur as part of a systemic lymphomatous process.

  b. It commonly occurs in the fifth and sixth decades.

  c. Some patients with AIDS have an aggressive form of lymphoma that predominantly involves the gastrointestinal tract. Patients who are immunosuppressed after organ transplant surgery are also at increased risk for lymphoma.

  d. The predominant site of involvement is the ileum.

2. Clinical features

  a. Fatigue, malaise, weight loss, and abdominal pain are the usual constitutional symptoms.

  b. Fever, night sweats, and pruritus do not typically occur in primary intestinal lymphoma. These symptoms are more typically associated with diffuse lymphoma.

  c. Some patients have symptoms of small bowel obstruction, perforation, or hemorrhage.

  d. Physical examination is usually unremarkable unless obstruction or bleeding is present. Diffuse lymphadenopathy does not usually occur in the primary intestinal form of lymphoma.

3. Diagnosis

  a. **Contrast radiography** may show submucosal nodularity, ulceration, or diffuse mucosal folds.

  b. CT scan is helpful for staging. It may show diffuse thickening of the wall of the small bowel.

4. Treatment

a. Most patients require **surgical exploration** for diagnosis, staging, and relief of the obstruction or perforation. Patients who have widespread disease may require surgery for bypass of an obstructing lesion.

b. If the tumor is localized, aggressive **surgical resection** in an attempt at cure improves the 5-year survival rate to 80%. When metastasis outside the regional nodes is present, death usually ensues within 1 year of surgery.

c. The survival benefit of adjuvant **chemoradiation therapy** is controversial. However, it is often used when the disease is believed to be systemic.

Ⅲ Meckel's Diverticulum

A. GENERAL CHARACTERISTICS

1. Meckel's diverticulum is the most common congenital anomaly of the gastrointestinal tract. It has an incidence of approximately 2% in the general population. Most people who have this condition remain asymptomatic. Approximately half of people who become symptomatic are younger than 2 years of age.

2. Meckel's diverticulum results from persistence of the embryonic yolk stalk. Typically, it arises from the antimesenteric border of the small bowel at the terminal ileum 40–50 cm proximal to the ileocecal valve in the adult.

3. The diverticulum may have ectopic gastric mucosa that may cause ulceration of the adjacent ileum.

B. CLINICAL FEATURES

1. Patients may have episodic gastrointestinal hemorrhage. The hemorrhage occurs when ectopic gastric mucosa within the diverticulum causes ulceration of the ileal mucosa. Usually, bleeding is red instead of melanotic because its origin is distal to the ligament of Treitz.

2. Small bowel obstruction may occur as a result of intussusception involving the diverticulum. It also may occur secondary to a volvulus around an adhesive band associated with the diverticulum.

3. If diverticulitis occurs, symptoms may mimic those of appendicitis. Unlike appendicitis, however, these symptoms may recur.

C. DIAGNOSIS

1. When the diagnosis of Meckel's diverticulum is suspected, a **pertechnetate radioisotope scan** may be diagnostic for patients who have ectopic gastric mucosa.

2. Because many patients have an obstruction or symptoms similar to those of appendicitis, the diagnosis is often made at **surgery**.

3. **CT scan** may identify an area of inflammation that involves the distal ileum.

D. TREATMENT

1. After symptoms occur, surgical intervention with simple excision of the diverticulum is indicated.

2. If significant inflammation is found, a segment of small bowel, including the diverticulum, can be resected. Primary anastomosis is safe.

3. In an **adult**, an asymptomatic Meckel's diverticulum is sometimes found incidentally at laparotomy for another indication. In this case, the diverticulum is usually left in place because the risk of it becoming symptomatic is roughly equal to the risk of complications associated with its resection (2%–3%). In a **child**, the risk of symptoms developing with time is slightly greater. Therefore, resection should be undertaken.

Chapter 5

Disorders of the Large Intestine

I Diverticular Disease

A. GENERAL CHARACTERISTICS

1. Patients may have **diverticulosis** (multiple diverticula) or **diverticulitis** (inflammation of the diverticula).
2. Most diverticula occur in the **sigmoid colon**. They are caused by increased pressure generated in this region of the colon. Diverticula are more common in people with low-fiber diets who have less stool bulk.
3. These diverticula tend to be **false diverticula** because they involve only the mucosa and submucosa, not all three layers of the bowel wall. The mucosa and submucosa herniate through the muscularis. They tend to herniate through weak points in the colonic wall, typically where mesenteric blood vessels penetrate the circular muscle layer.
4. Diverticulitis is caused by **impaction** of **feces** within a diverticulum. This impaction causes obstruction and leads to infection.
5. The **incidence** of diverticular disease increases with age. Diverticula are present in 30%–50% of people older than 50 years of age, but only 25% of these people have symptoms.

B. CLINICAL FEATURES

1. Diverticulosis alone does not produce pain. However, the diverticula are prone to hemorrhage and can cause significant lower gastrointestinal bleeding.
2. **Diverticulitis** usually causes fever and lower abdominal pain.
   a. Tachycardia and hypotension usually occur with significant diverticulitis, which is often associated with perforation or abscess formation with sepsis.
   b. Guarding and percussion tenderness over the left lower quadrant are common. Diffuse abdominal tenderness and guarding or a rigid abdomen indicates free perforation.
   c. Tenderness may be noted on rectal examination. Fullness may also be appreciated and may be caused by an abscess or phlegmonous inflammation. Stool is usually negative for occult blood.
   d. If there is significant inflammation or abscess formation, colonic obstruction may occur. Obstruction is indicated by increasing abdominal distension and reduced or absent bowel function. Vomiting may also be present.
   e. If a colovesical fistula develops secondary to the infection, patients may have pneumaturia (air in the urine stream) and dysuria. A colovaginal fistula may also occur, leading to stool from the vagina. Colocutaneous fistula may also occur.

C. DIAGNOSIS

1. **Lower gastrointestinal hemorrhage associated with diverticulosis** is usually diagnosed by **colonoscopy**. If bleeding obscures endoscopic visualization, **angiography** can identify the portion of the colon that is bleeding.

2. A **computed tomography (CT) scan** usually diagnoses **acute diverticulitis**. This scan shows inflammatory changes in the sigmoid colon. It may also show sites of abscess, obstruction, fistula, or perforation. Patients who have acute diverticulitis should not undergo colonoscopy until symptoms subside because of the risk of producing perforation (if it is not already present) as a result of insufflation of the colon.

3. **Barium enema** can be used to diagnose **diverticulosis** in **asymptomatic** patients. Barium should not be used in patients who have symptoms because barium peritonitis may occur if perforation is present. **Gastrografin enema** can be used to verify suspected **obstruction** (Figure 5-1). Typically, this test is not a sensitive means to identify a colovesical fistula.

4. A **white blood cell count** usually shows leukocytosis, although it may not be present in mild cases.

D. TREATMENT

1. **Bleeding diverticulosis** can often be managed supportively with blood **transfusion**. Most hemorrhage stops spontaneously.

   a. Patients who require more than 6 units of blood or who are hemodynamically unstable despite resuscitative efforts should undergo surgical resection. Similarly, a patient who has had more than one episode of diverticular hemorrhage in the past is at significantly increased risk of rebleeding. Elective surgical resection is needed before rebleeding occurs.

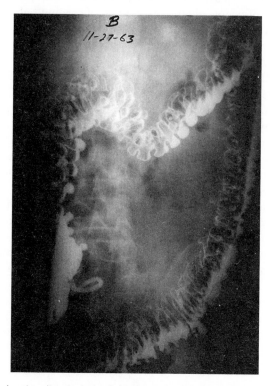

● **Figure 5.1** Barium enema showing diverticulosis of the sigmoid colon. The diverticula are the multiple pouches off the colon.

b.   If the bleeding site is localized by endoscopy or angiography, **partial colon resection** of the bleeding segment with **primary anastomosis** can be performed (usually sigmoid resection). If the site is not localized, **abdominal colectomy** must be performed to ensure that the site of bleeding is removed (Figure 5-2).

2. **Uncomplicated diverticulitis** (absence of perforation, obstruction, fistula, or abscess) often responds to **antibiotics, bowel rest,** and **intravenous fluid administration.** Antibiotics that cover *Escherichia coli* and *Bacteroides* species are most often used (e.g., a second-generation cephalosporin in combination with metronidazole).

3. **Partial obstruction** as a result of **severe phlegmonous inflammation** of **acute diverticulitis** may resolve with **bowel rest** and **antibiotics.**
    a.   If the symptoms of obstruction do not improve or if the obstruction is complete, **partial colectomy** of the diseased segment is indicated.
    b.   In the acute setting, a **Hartmann's procedure** is indicated (partial colectomy with closure of the distal rectal stump and proximal colostomy). This procedure is used because there is a significant risk of anastomotic breakdown when the colon and surrounding tissues are acutely inflamed and infected.

4. **Peridiverticular abscess** can be treated with **CT-guided aspiration.** If complete drainage is achieved and the patient responds to antibiotics and bowel rest, an **elective partial colon resection** should be performed 3–6 months after the episode to prevent recurrence. This approach allows time for inflammation to subside and permits a resection with primary anastomosis (one-stage procedure) rather than a temporary colostomy. Patients who have a temporary colostomy require a second procedure to restore intestinal continuity.

5. **More than one episode** of **uncomplicated diverticulitis** is an indication for **elective sigmoid resection.** The risk of further episodes and complications increases with each attack.

6. **Fistula** requires surgical repair with excision of the sigmoid colon. Preoperatively, the patient should undergo bowel preparation with **oral antibiotics** (e.g., erythromycin and neomycin) and **Fleet enema.** If inflammation is minimal and adequate

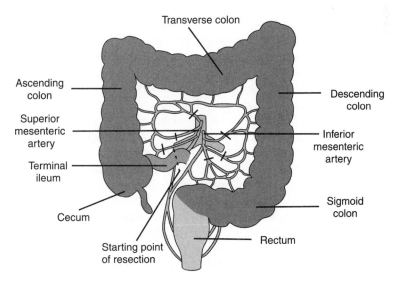

● **Figure 5.2** Total abdominal colectomy for bleeding diverticulosis. When the bleeding diverticula cannot be localized to a specific segment, the colon is removed from the cecum to the rectum. The arterial branches from the superior mesenteric artery that supply the ascending and transverse colon are divided, as are the branches from the inferior mesenteric artery that supply the descending and sigmoid colon. An ileorectal anastomosis is then performed.

bowel preparation is achieved, **a primary anastomosis** may be attempted. If significant inflammation is present, the fistula should be repaired and a **Hartmann's procedure** performed. A procedure to restore intestinal continuity should be performed 3–6 months after the resection.

7. **Uncomplicated diverticulitis** that does not resolve with **medical therapy** (persistent leukocytosis with pain that does not improve after 48–72 hours of optimal antibiotics) is an indication for **Hartmann's procedure.**

8. **Sepsis** and evidence of **perforation** requires **rapid resuscitation** and prompt Hartmann's procedure.

Ⅱ Colonic Neoplasms

A. GENERAL CHARACTERISTICS

1. The incidence of colonic neoplasms increases steadily with age from the second decade to the ninth decade. However, these neoplasms are most likely to occur between the sixth and eighth decades.

2. Elevated fat intake and low fiber intake are associated with an increased risk of colorectal cancer.

3. Tumor development is a multistep process. It begins with the growth of a benign adenomatous polyp that transforms into a malignancy.

4. Several **genetic alterations** are linked to the development of these tumors:
   a. Mutation of the K-*ras* proto-oncogene. This gene is responsible for the production of G protein, which is important for proliferative signal transduction.
   b. Loss of the adenomatous polyposis coli (APC) gene. This cell growth suppressor gene is found on the long arm of chromosome 5.
   c. Alteration of the p53 gene. This tumor suppressor gene is the most commonly isolated genetic abnormality in colorectal tumors.
   d. Allelic loss of the "deleted in colorectal carcinoma" gene (DCC). This gene is important for cell recognition and adhesion.

5. Another family of genetic mutations is associated with a specific form of colorectal carcinoma known as hereditary nonpolyposis colorectal carcinoma (HNPCC). These genes (*hMSH1* and *hMSH2*) are involved in DNA repair. This group of patients accounts for 5%–10% of colorectal tumors. There are two forms of HNPCC: Lynch syndrome I and Lynch syndrome II.
   a. **Lynch syndrome I** is characterized by colorectal tumors that usually occur in the right side of the colon (most tumors occur in the left). These tumors also occur at an earlier age than most tumors (30–50 years). Lynch syndrome I is transmitted as an autosomal dominant trait.
   b. **Lynch syndrome II** is similar to Lynch syndrome I, but these patients also have early-onset carcinoma of the endometrium, ovaries, or stomach.

6. Ulcerative colitis and, to a lesser extent, Crohn's disease are associated with an increased risk of colorectal cancer. In approximately 3% of patients with ulcerative colitis, a colorectal malignancy develops within the first 10 years of the disease. In an additional 20%, a malignancy develops in the next 10 years.

7. **Polyps** are associated with an increased risk of malignancy of the colon.
   a. Nonneoplastic polyps have no malignant potential. These include hamartoma, inflammatory, juvenile, and hyperplastic polyps, as classified histologically.
   b. Neoplastic polyps are known as adenomas. They have malignant potential or may already be malignant at diagnosis. There are three kinds of adenomas:
      i. **Tubular adenoma** is the most common polyp and constitutes 75% of all neoplastic polyps. Invasive malignancies are seen in 5% of these adenomas.

ii.   **Tubulovillous adenoma** constitutes 15% of all neoplastic polyps. Invasive malignancies are seen in 20% of these adenomas.

iii. **Villous adenoma** constitutes 10% of all neoplastic polyps. Invasive malignancies are seen in 40% of these adenomas.

B. CLINICAL FEATURES

1. Intermittent abdominal discomfort, nausea, or vomiting may be present, but these symptoms are nonspecific. Patients who have an obstructing tumor have vomiting, hyperactive bowel sounds, abdominal distension, and absence of bowel function. Peritonitis with guarding and fever indicates a perforation of the tumor-associated bowel.

2. **Bleeding.** Gross blood may be the first presenting sign. Bright red blood per rectum is typically associated with left-sided lesions. Melena is usually associated with right-sided lesions. Tests for fecal occult blood are often positive.

3. A palpable abdominal mass may be present.

4. Rectal tumors may cause tenesmus and may even be palpable on digital rectal examination.

5. In advanced cases, a metastatic liver mass (the most common site of metastasis for colorectal cancer) may be palpable. Weight loss may be noted. Lung metastasis also occurs, usually after liver metastasis.

C. DIAGNOSIS

1. **Digital rectal examination** may show a palpable rectal tumor.

2. **Flexible sigmoidoscopy** allows visualization of the distal 35–65 cm of colon and permits biopsy of lesions. This procedure may be therapeutic for small polyps that have evidence of malignancy in situ.

3. Patients who have symptoms can be evaluated in one of two ways.

    a. **Double-contrast barium enema** allows visualization of the intra-abdominal colon. This technique can detect polyps or tumors as small as 0.5–1.0 cm. However, because it provides poor visualization of the rectosigmoid colon, it should be supplemented with flexible sigmoidoscopy.

    b. **Colonoscopy** can be used instead of barium enema and flexible sigmoidoscopy, but it requires more skill. Complications that require surgical intervention (e.g., perforation, hemorrhage) occur in 0.1%–0.3% of cases.

4. **Carcinoembryonic antigen** is an effective marker in detecting tumor recurrence. However, it is insensitive as a primary screening tool for the disease.

5. **Screening.** Beginning at 50 years of age, patients who have no significant risk factors should undergo routine screening that includes yearly fecal occult blood testing and digital rectal examination. These patients should also undergo flexible sigmoidoscopy every 3–5 years.

D. STAGING AND PROGNOSIS

1. Factors associated with a **poor prognosis** include poorly differentiated tumors, mucinous-producing tumors, and vascular or lymphatic invasion.

2. The **Astler-Coller staging system** defines the local and metastatic extent of the tumor. This stage is of clinical importance because it affects prognosis and dictates subsequent therapy.

    a. **Stage A** tumors invade the mucosa only. The 5-year survival rate after resection is 90%.

    b. **Stage B** tumors invade through the mucosa but have **no lymph node involvement.** The 5-year survival rate for all stage B tumors after resection is 75%.

        i.   **Stage B_1** tumors invade into the muscularis propria.

        ii.   **Stage B_2** tumors invade the serosa but not adjacent organs.

        iii. **Stage B_3** tumors invade through the serosa and involve adjacent organs.

    c.   **Stage C_{1-3} tumors** have identical tumor invasion as for stages B_{1-3} but **with lymph node involvement.** The 5-year survival rate for all stage C tumors after resection is 50%.

    d.   **Stage D** tumors have distant organ metastasis. The 5-year survival rate is less than 10%.

E. TREATMENT

1. **Polyps can be removed endoscopically.** If histologic examination identifies a malignancy that does not penetrate the muscularis mucosa, no further treatment is necessary. If invasion of the muscularis mucosa occurs, partial colectomy and lymph node removal is advised.

2. **Surgical excision.** The goal of surgery is to remove the tumor mass and involved adjacent tissue along with the paracolonic lymph nodes. To reduce the risk of local recurrence, the margin of colon resection should be 5 cm both proximally and distally. Preoperative bowel preparation includes enema and either ingestion of a hyperosmolar liquid or an erythromycin/neomycin regimen the day before surgery to minimize contamination during the resection.

3. **Primary anastomosis** is usually feasible if there is no evidence of intra-abdominal infection as a result of perforation. Colonic anastomoses must be tension free and have an adequate blood supply. Otherwise, they are at risk for breakdown and subsequent leak, which can cause intra-abdominal and systemic sepsis.

4. Right colon tumors are usually resected by a **right hemicolectomy.** Tumors of the hepatic flexure are resected by an extended right hemicolectomy to include the proximal transverse colon.

5. Tumors of the left colon are resected with a **left hemicolectomy.** Splenic flexure tumors can be resected with an extended left hemicolectomy to include the distal transverse colon.

6. Sigmoid tumors and tumors that involve the upper third of the rectum can be resected by a **low anterior resection,** which removes the rectosigmoid colon.

7. Low rectal tumors that are less than 7–8 cm from the anal verge generally cannot be removed without removing the sphincters to get an adequate margin of at least 2 cm distal to the tumor. In such cases, an abdominoperineal resection (resection of the anus and rectum with colostomy) may be required. Alternatively, if a tumor is borderline in terms of the ability to remove it and spare the sphincters, neoadjuvant chemoradiation with 5-fluorouracil (5-FU) has reduced tumor size, making it possible to resect via a low anterior approach.

8. **Hepatic resection.** Resection of an isolated single hepatic metastasis can increase the 5-year survival rate to 30%. Therefore, this procedure is advisable in patients who have no other medical contraindication to a significant hepatic resection.

9. **Radiation therapy in conjunction with surgery** reduces the risk of local recurrence. Radiation therapy is used only for rectal tumors because these tumors have a higher incidence of local recurrence than other colonic neoplasms. Further, it is difficult to radiate other parts of the colon without causing significant radiation damage to the small bowel and adjacent organs.

10. **Chemotherapy** with 5-FU and leucovorin improves the 5-year survival rate.

Ⅲ Colonic Volvulus

A. GENERAL CHARACTERISTICS

1. Colonic volvulus is caused by **twisting** of the intestine around its mesenteric axis. It often leads to obstruction.

2. Either the sigmoid colon (80%) or the cecum (20%) may be involved.
   a. **Sigmoid volvulus** occurs in the elderly, in patients who have neurologic or psychiatric disorders, and in those who have chronic constipation or who abuse laxatives.
   b. **Cecal volvulus** is caused by incomplete peritoneal fixation of the right colon during fetal development. It can occur at any age.

B. **CLINICAL FEATURES**
   1. **Sigmoid volvulus**
      a. Abdominal distension (typical)
      b. Crampy abdominal pain
      c. Constipation or absence of bowel function or flatus
      d. Nausea and vomiting with dehydration
      e. Mild abdominal tenderness
      f. Peritoneal signs, fever, and tachycardia (indications of colonic ischemia or infarction)
      g. No stool on rectal examination
   2. **Cecal volvulus**
      a. Crampy abdominal pain with distension
      b. Nausea and vomiting with distension
      c. Peritoneal signs, fever, and tachycardia (indications of bowel ischemia)
      d. Absence of bowel function or flatus

C. **DIAGNOSIS**
   1. An elevated white cell count suggests bowel ischemia.
   2. **Plain radiographs**
      a. **Sigmoid volvulus.** Plain radiographs show dilated sigmoid colon arising from the pelvis (**bent inner tube sign**). Large bowel dilation proximal to the sigmoid volvulus may be present (Figure 5-3A).
      b. **Cecal volvulus.** Plain radiographs show dilated small bowel and a dilated cecum with air–fluid levels.
   3. **Barium enema** shows narrowing at the point of the volvulus (see Figure 5-3B).

D. **TREATMENT**
   1. If strangulation is not present (no peritonitis), **rigid sigmoidoscopy** can reduce the volvulus. A rectal tube is left in place beyond the point of obstruction to prevent immediate recurrence. If necrosis is seen on sigmoidoscopy, **low anterior resection** is required to remove the affected segment.
   2. After reduction, medically fit patients should undergo elective sigmoid resection because the recurrence rate for volvulus is 50%–90%.
   3. If sigmoidoscopy does not reduce the volvulus (10% of patients), **surgical reduction** is necessary. The bowel should not be removed during the first operation unless it is necrotic. Unprepared bowel carries an increased risk of anastomotic leak if resection is performed. If necrotic bowel is found, a sigmoid resection with colostomy and stapling of the rectal stump should be performed (**Hartmann's procedure**).
   4. Cecal volvulus necessitates operative intervention. **Resection of necrotic bowel with primary anastomosis** is usually feasible (unlike sigmoid volvulus), even in unprepared bowel. To prevent recurrence, a right hemicolectomy with primary anastomosis can be performed with low morbidity.

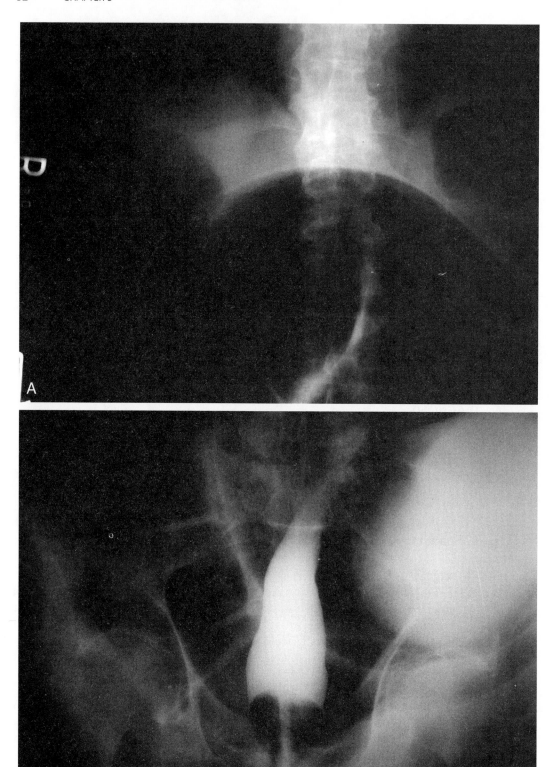

● **Figure 5.3** (*A*) Plain abdominal film showing a sigmoid volvulus. The classic bent inner tube sign is present, representing a closed-loop obstruction of the sigmoid colon. (*B*) Barium enema showing a sigmoid volvulus. The colon tapers to the obstructed segment, suggesting a twist in the colon.

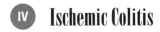

Ischemic Colitis

A. GENERAL CHARACTERISTICS

1. Ischemic colitis usually occurs in patients who are older than 50 years of age. It often requires a high index of suspicion because symptoms may be subtle. Ischemic colitis may be **transient** (most common), may cause **strictures**, or may lead to **gangrenous injury**.

2. Ischemic colitis has two broad etiologies: **arterial occlusive disease** and **nonocclusive disease**.
   a. **Occlusive disease** includes thromboembolism (a mural thrombus caused by atrial fibrillation embolizes to the intestinal vessel), thrombosis of an intestinal vessel, vascular compression secondary to neoplasm, and vasculitis.
   b. **Nonocclusive disease** causes ischemia as a result of a low-flow state. This state causes poor colonic perfusion and includes hypovolemia, cardiac dysfunction, and drugs that increase splanchnic vascular tone (e.g., vasopressin).

B. CLINICAL FEATURES

1. Ischemic colitis classically causes **abrupt** onset of abdominal pain (usually in the left lower quadrant) with bloody diarrhea (hematochezia or melena).
2. Nausea and vomiting may be present.
3. Abdominal tenderness is not always present. It is often a late sign that occurs after ischemia causes necrosis.
4. Fever and tachycardia usually do not occur until necrosis and perforation develop.

C. DIAGNOSIS

1. **Leukocytosis** may be present when necrosis begins.
2. **Arterial blood gas** measurements may show metabolic acidosis (anion gap). However, this finding is not always present.
3. **Upright chest films** may show free air under the diaphragm if perforation occurs as a result of necrosis.
4. An **abdominal series** may show pneumatosis intestinalis (air within the bowel wall) or portal vein air. These are signs of invasion of gas-forming organisms.
5. **CT scan** may show a thickened bowel wall or occlusion of the superior mesenteric artery.
6. **Colonoscopy** is the most useful diagnostic modality because it can identify ischemic mucosa before frank necrosis occurs. The procedure must be done carefully and with minimal insufflation because an ischemic colon can perforate easily.
7. **Barium enema** is no longer indicated because it precludes colonoscopy.
8. **Arteriography** usually is not beneficial unless a patient is suspected to have superior mesenteric artery occlusion that causes small bowel and right colon ischemia. In this case, a vascular procedure may be necessary.

D. TREATMENT

1. **Transient ischemic colitis**
   a. If the injury is reversible and the patient has no signs of peritonitis that suggest full-thickness ischemia or perforation, complete healing is typical.
   b. If ileus is present, **nasogastric suction** should be performed.
   c. **Bowel rest** and **oxygen supplementation** are required. **Intravenous rehydration** should also be provided to optimize flow to the ischemic areas.
   d. **Broad-spectrum antibiotics** to cover coliforms, anaerobes, and enterococci (e.g., a second- or third-generation cephalosporin and metronidazole) should be administered.

      e.   Patients whose condition worsens with this therapy have progressed to gangrenous colitis and are at risk for perforation. In this case, surgical intervention is needed (see below).

2. Chronic ischemic colitis

      a.   After the initial ischemic event, a stricture may develop and cause obstruction. Patients may also have persistent pain as a result of chronic segmental ischemia (2% of patients). These patients require **elective surgery** to remove the diseased segment with reanastomosis of the remaining normal colon.

      b.   **Annual colonoscopy** is recommended for patients who are asymptomatic but have stricture or persistent ischemia on follow-up colonoscopy. Surgery is not required unless symptoms occur.

3. Gangrenous colitis

      a.   Patients who have gangrenous colitis are in shock. They require **rapid volume replacement, emergent surgery,** and broad-spectrum intravenous antibiotics. There is **no time for bowel preparation,** and preparation may lead to perforation (if it has not already occurred).

      b.   The intraoperative appearance of the serosal surface of the colon can be misleading. **Significant mucosal necrosis may occur without serosal change.** Palpation of pulses in the mesentery, Doppler signals, and Wood's lamp visualization with fluorescein injection are useful methods to identify poorly perfused segments and plan resection.

      c.   In most cases, an **end colostomy** and **mucous fistula** of the distal bowel should be performed. This approach eliminates the risk of anastomotic leak, which is likely in the septic patient who has a diseased colon. Further, it permits direct visualization of the bowel to assess ongoing ischemia.

      d.   If there is any question about bowel viability at the initial operation, a second-look operation should be performed in 24 hours. Second-look surgery should be performed sooner if the sepsis appears to worsen despite adequate resuscitation.

Ⓥ Appendicitis

A. GENERAL CHARACTERISTICS. Appendicitis is caused by obstruction of the appendiceal orifice with inspissated fecal material. The obstruction increases intraluminal pressure and causes ischemia of the appendiceal wall, subsequent necrosis, and eventual perforation. Appendicitis is common in children and adolescents.

B. CLINICAL FEATURES

  1. The **classic presentation** includes fever, nausea and vomiting, and abdominal pain.

  2. Pain is initially **periumbilical** and progresses to the right lower quadrant at McBurney's point (Figure 5-4). Pain usually precedes nausea and vomiting.

  3. If nausea, vomiting, and diarrhea are the predominant symptoms, **gastroenteritis** is the more likely diagnosis.

  4. Tenderness and eventually guarding are present at **McBurney's point.**

  5. The **psoas sign** (pain with extension of the right hip) or the **obturator sign** may be present (pain with internal rotation and flexion of the thigh).

  6. **Rectal examination** may elicit tenderness in the right pelvis. This area may be palpable if perforation with abscess is present.

  7. If gross perforation occurs, **diffuse guarding and tenderness** may be noted. The patient will have significant tachycardia, fever, and possibly hypotension.

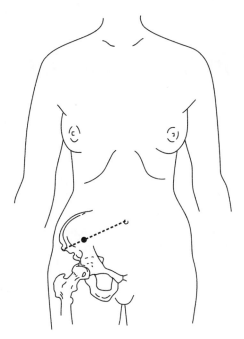

● **Figure 5.4** McBurney's point is located two-thirds the distance from the umbilicus to the anterior superior iliac spine. This site is most often localized to the area of greatest tenderness.

C. DIAGNOSIS

1. The **white cell count** is often elevated. However, a normal white cell count does not exclude the diagnosis.
2. **Plain abdominal films** may show a fecalith in the appendix in the right lower quadrant (10%–20% of patients).
3. **Ultrasound** may show an enlarged appendix (diameter >9 mm). Associated tenderness over the area carries an 80%–95% sensitivity. The absence of an identifiable appendix on ultrasound does not exclude the diagnosis.
4. **CT scan** may be used if the diagnosis is in question. It is also useful in older patients whose differential diagnosis includes colonic neoplasm.

D. TREATMENT

1. **Fluid resuscitation** should be initiated quickly in preparation for emergent laparotomy and appendectomy.
2. In unperforated appendicitis, a **second- or third-generation cephalosporin** usually provides adequate coverage and is required only perioperatively.
3. In perforated appendicitis, an **antibiotic regimen** covering *E. coli, Pseudomonas, Enterococcus,* and *Bacteroides* is necessary (e.g., ampicillin, gentamicin, metronidazole).
4. At **surgery**, if appendiceal perforation and abscess are present, the appendix is removed and the abscess drained. **Drains** should be left in place if there is significant intra-abdominal sepsis. The skin should be left open because there is a significant risk of wound infection postoperatively.
5. If the appendix is normal, it should be removed to eliminate it as a diagnostic possibility if symptoms recur. A **thorough exploration** for other causes should be performed (e.g., Meckel's diverticulum, tubo-ovarian abscess, diverticulitis, carcinoma).

Chapter 6

Inflammatory Bowel Disorders

I Ulcerative Colitis

A. GENERAL CHARACTERISTICS
1. Ulcerative colitis affects patients in youth or early middle age.
2. In ulcerative colitis, ulceration involves the mucosa and submucosa of the colon and rectum. The lesions are not transmural, as in Crohn's disease.
3. The cause is unknown, but a combination of infectious and environmental triggers associated with an autoimmune response may be involved.
4. The risk of colon cancer steadily increases 2% per year every year after the 10th year of disease.

B. CLINICAL FEATURES
1. Patients often have bloody diarrhea, abdominal pain and tenderness, weight loss, and pallor.
2. The disease may progress to fulminant colitis with diffuse abdominal guarding, distension, fever, and bloody diarrhea as a result of toxic megacolon.
3. Extraintestinal manifestations include inflammation of the ocular components, lower extremity arthralgia, pyoderma gangrenosum, hepatitis, biliary cirrhosis, and sclerosing cholangitis.

C. DIAGNOSIS
1. Ulcerative colitis has no pathognomonic laboratory, radiographic, or histologic features. Infectious causes of bloody diarrhea must be excluded, including stool sample cultures for *Campylobacter, Salmonella, Escherichia coli,* ameba, and *Clostridium difficile.*
2. Flexible sigmoidoscopy shows friable hemorrhagic mucosa. Severe disease may cause ulceration and purulent exudate. Unlike the skip lesions seen in Crohn's disease, the associated lesions are continuous. Also unlike Crohn's disease, the rectum is often involved.
3. Barium enema may show a diffuse granular appearance. In patients who have more severe disease, the disappearance of haustra and loss of colonic redundancy and caliber may be noted. Patients who have toxic megacolon should not undergo barium enema because of the risk of perforation.

D. TREATMENT
1. **Medications.** Sulfasalazine is effective in treating mild to moderate disease. Steroid therapy is beneficial for chronic disease and acute flares. Azathioprine and 6-mercaptopurine may be effective when sulfasalazine and steroids are not.
2. **Total proctocolectomy** is indicated for patients who have intractable disease that does not improve with medical management, those who have fulminant colitis that

causes toxic megacolon or continuous hemorrhage, those who have colonic obstruction as a result of stricture, and those who are suspected to have cancer.

3. In the **emergency** setting, **subtotal colectomy with ileostomy** is the procedure of choice because there is a substantial risk of anastomotic leak during the period of acute toxicity. Elective subtotal colectomy with ileorectal anastomosis is not an ideal approach because it leaves behind the rectum, which is prone to recurrent disease and malignancy in 15%–25% of patients. Although proctocolectomy with ileostomy was used in the past, currently, the formation of an **ileal pouch** with **ileoanal anastomosis** is considered the procedure of choice in the elective setting (Figure 6-1). A diverting temporary loop ileostomy is constructed proximal to the pouch anastomosis to prevent leak until the anastomosis heals.

Ⅱ Crohn's Disease

A. GENERAL CHARACTERISTICS

1. Crohn's disease causes chronic transmural inflammation. It can involve any portion of the intestine, from the mouth to the anus. The ileocecal area is most often involved. The disease may have an indolent course, with periods of acute exacerbation, or it may be fulminant.

2. Crohn's disease usually occurs in patients who are 15–30 years old. A second peak incidence occurs in the sixth decade.

3. The etiology is unknown, but infectious and autoimmune factors are believed to be involved.

4. The lesions involve mucosal ulceration with granuloma, fissure, and fistula formation. Fistulas may form between loops of bowel or may involve any other organ, including skin.

B. CLINICAL FEATURES

1. Patients with Crohn's disease have colicky abdominal pain, diarrhea, anorexia, nausea, and vomiting. Patients with stricture have symptoms of bowel obstruction, including decreased bowel movements, abdominal distension, and vomiting.

2. Patients with Crohn's disease may have a propensity to renal calculi because of the formation of oxalate stones.

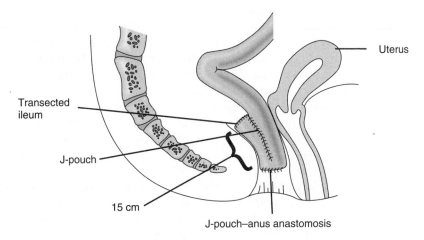

● **Figure 6.1** The J-pouch ileoanal anastomosis after proctocolectomy. The hook of the J-pouch is opened and anastomosed to the anus. The pouch acts as a reservoir.

3. Intra-abdominal infection may occur as a result of fistula and abscess formation. It may lead to peritoneal findings, fever, leukocytosis, and even sepsis.

4. Anal involvement is common and causes recurrent fistulas, fissures, and perirectal abscesses.

5. Toxic megacolon may occur and cause diffuse abdominal tenderness, distension, and sepsis.

6. Extraintestinal manifestations include ocular inflammation, arthralgia, pyoderma gangrenosum, and sclerosing cholangitis.

7. Less commonly, patients may have free perforation with generalized peritonitis and sepsis. Occasionally, the ulcerating lesions cause significant gastrointestinal hemorrhage.

C. DIAGNOSIS

1. No specific laboratory test is diagnostic for Crohn's disease. However, chronic anemia, hypoalbuminemia, and leukocytosis are common.

2. A barium small bowel series may show cobblestoning, strictures, and skip lesions.

3. Colonoscopy permits biopsy of the affected areas and assessment of the extent of disease. The presence of skip lesions, cobblestoning, and aphthous ulcers differentiates Crohn's disease from ulcerative colitis.

4. Computed tomography (CT) scan is useful in diagnosing intra-abdominal abscess.

D. TREATMENT

1. Opiates are often necessary to control pain and improve the symptoms of diarrhea.

2. Acute exacerbations may require bowel rest and total parenteral nutrition.

3. Steroids, sulfasalazine, azathioprine, and 6-mercaptopurine are effective in reducing symptoms and inducing remission. Broad-spectrum antibiotics are required for septic complications.

4. Surgical excision of diseased segments is not curative, and recurrence is typical. Surgery is reserved for patients who have complications of Crohn's disease, with the intent to preserve as much bowel as possible.

   a. **Fistula management.** When fistulas lead to infectious complications or high output, surgical management is required. Resection of the fistula and the diseased bowel segment is required. In a medically stable patient, a fistula associated with intra-abdominal abscess is best treated initially with CT-guided drainage of the abscess and antibiotic therapy. Once the abdomen is sterilized, the fistulous tract and the affected segment can be surgically resected with a primary anastomosis without fear of leakage because of a septic environment.

   b. **Stricture management.** For short strictures that cause bowel obstruction, stricturoplasty rather than resection should be performed. Recurrent resections result in short-gut syndrome. Multiple strictures in close proximity may be best treated with resection of the isolated segment.

   c. **Colonic involvement.** Proctocolectomy with ileostomy is the procedure of choice for patients who have toxic megacolon or diffuse colonic involvement with unrelenting symptoms. If the rectum is spared and unrelenting colonic involvement is present without overt sepsis or toxic megacolon, resection with ileorectal anastomosis is feasible.

   d. **Anal involvement.** Patients who have a simple fistula can be treated with fistulotomy. However, complex fistulas are usually transsphincteric, and radical fistulotomy would destroy the sphincter. In this case, the best approach is conservative partial excision, fistulotomy, and drainage.

Chapter 7

Disorders of the Rectum and Anus

I. Anal Fistula and Perianal Abscess

A. GENERAL CHARACTERISTICS

1. **Perianal abscess** occurs when an anal gland becomes obstructed and causes bacterial overgrowth and suppuration. Other causes include carcinoma, Crohn's disease, radiation (which produces scarring and fibrosis that can obstruct the anal gland), and the presence of a foreign body.

2. **Anal fistula.** The abscess usually drains through a fistula, or tract, between the opening in the anal gland and an external opening. Anal fistulas may be intersphincteric, transsphincteric, suprasphincteric, or extrasphincteric.

3. **Drainage.** The abscess usually drains in the intersphincteric space, down into the perianal area. If the infection spreads through the external sphincter, it causes an **ischiorectal abscess.** Occasionally, transsphincteric extension in the posterior midline causes a postanal space abscess that extends into the ischiorectal space unilaterally or bilaterally. This extension produces a **horseshoe abscess** (Figure 7-1).

B. CLINICAL FEATURES

1. **Perianal abscess** usually begins with a dull ache in the perianal area. Severe pain, tenesmus, and constipation with fever quickly develop. If the abscess extends to the perianal space, induration, erythema, or fluctuance may occur. However, because the subcutaneous tissue in the perianal area is abundant, these signs may not be prominent. Digital rectal examination elicits tenderness.

2. **Anal fistula** causes intermittent or persistent purulent discharge from a perianal opening. Induration and scarring often occur around the opening. Patients may have a history of perianal abscess.

C. DIAGNOSIS

1. With **perianal abscess**, leukocytosis is often present. The diagnosis is typically made on clinical grounds.

2. With **anal fistula**, no specific laboratory abnormality is noted unless the patient also has Crohn's disease (see Chapter 6).

D. TREATMENT

1. **Perianal abscess**
   a. Incision and drainage is the mainstay of treatment. The administration of antibiotics alone is suboptimal and may permit further extension and sepsis.
   b. A cruciate incision near the anal verge over the fluctuant area provides drainage. If a fistula occurs between the drainage site and the cavity, the resulting fistulotomy wound is shorter.

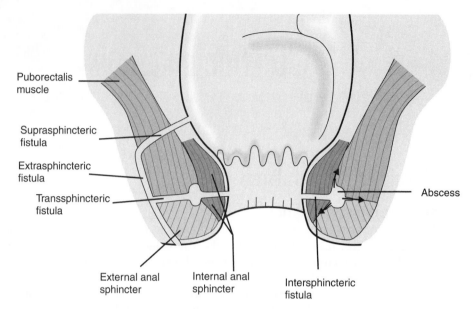

Puborectalis
muscle

Suprasphincteric
fistula

Extrasphincteric
fistula

Transsphincteric
fistula

Abscess

External anal
sphincter

Internal anal
sphincter

Intersphincteric
fistula

● **Figure 7.1** Perianal abscess channels can be intersphincteric, extrasphincteric, transsphincteric, or suprasphincteric.

2. **Anal fistula**

   a. Adequate fistulotomy requires identification of the internal opening. **Goodsall's rule** dictates that external openings anterior to the transverse anal line lead to an internal opening in a radial fashion. Posterior external openings lead to an internal opening, typically in the posterior midline. Once the tract is open, it closes from the base up.

   b. During fistulotomy, care must be taken not to induce incontinence. The tract usually passes below the puborectalis muscle. Incontinence after fistulotomy is unlikely if care is taken to preserve the external sphincter and puborectalis muscles.

   c. Patients who have a history of mild incontinence may become completely incontinent after fistulotomy. These patients will do better with an **anal Seton**. This procedure involves placing a suture or tie through the tract and tying it snugly to produce local ischemia and scarring. The patient is reevaluated weekly, and a tighter Seton is placed. Eventually, scarring of the tract occurs from the base up to the skin. The scarring preserves continence.

Ⅱ Anal Fissure

A. GENERAL CHARACTERISTICS

1. Anal fissures affect people of any age. Anal fissure is the most common cause of rectal bleeding in infants.

2. An anal fissure is caused by a linear tear in the anoderm. The tear may be located in the posterior (90%) or the anterior midline (10%). The passage of a large, hard stool typically causes the fissure.

3. Fissures may be associated with Crohn's disease, ulcerative colitis, AIDS, syphilis, or tuberculosis.

4. The tenuous blood supply in the posterior midline is believed to account for the predominance of posterior midline fissures.

5. Pain associated with the tear increases anal sphincter tone and spasm, precludes healing of the torn mucosa, and worsens pain.

6. Acute anal fissure is a partial-thickness tear. Chronic anal fissure persists and is a full-thickness tear that exposes the circular fibers of the internal anal sphincter.

B. CLINICAL FEATURES
1. Acute pain occurs on defecation (tenesmus).
2. The patient may report a small amount of bleeding on the tissue paper after a bowel movement.
3. Inspection usually shows a tear in the posterior midline between the anal verge and the dentate line. The patient cannot tolerate a digital rectal examination. If the diagnosis is made by inspection, a digital examination should not be performed. After the fissure heals, a complete examination should be performed.
4. A sentinel pile (Figure 7-2) may occur with chronic fissures.

C. DIAGNOSIS is made on clinical grounds.

D. TREATMENT
1. **Acute anal fissure**
   a. Acute anal fissures resolve with conservative therapy. **Sitz baths** after each bowel movement help to relieve discomfort. **Topical anesthetic agents** also reduce discomfort. These agents reduce spasm and permit healing.
   b. **Stool bulking agents** reduce discomfort and prevent recurrence.
   c. **Nitroglycerin paste** applied to the area improves healing rates by enhancing smooth muscle relaxation of the internal anal sphincter. Healing typically occurs in 2–4 weeks.
2. **Chronic anal fissure.** When a fissure does not respond to medical therapy and becomes chronic, surgical therapy is warranted. Lateral internal anal sphincterotomy can be performed under local or light general anesthesia. The intersphincteric groove is palpated, and a no. 11 blade is inserted into this space on the right or left side. The blade is rotated 90° and then removed. Care is taken not to cut the anoderm. The blade incises the internal sphincter and releases the spasm, allowing the

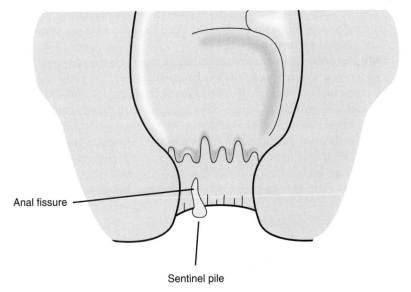

Anal fissure

Sentinel pile

● **Figure 7.2** The sentinel pile is a tag that is often associated with an anal fissure.

anoderm to heal. Because the external anal sphincter is maintained, the rate of incontinence is relatively low (3%). The recurrence rate is approximately 10%.

Ⅲ Hemorrhoids

A. GENERAL CHARACTERISTICS
1. Hemorrhoids often occur in pregnant women, but they can occur in anyone at any age.
2. Hemorrhoids may be external (distal to the dentate line) or internal. Internal hemorrhoids are classified according to the degree of prolapse.
   a. **First-degree** hemorrhoids cause painless bleeding with no prolapse.
   b. **Second-degree** hemorrhoids are spontaneously reducible and prolapse with defecation.
   c. **Third-degree** hemorrhoids cause prolapse that requires manual reduction.
   d. **Fourth-degree** hemorrhoids cause irreducible prolapse.
3. Hemorrhoids are most commonly located in the left lateral, right anterior, and right posterior positions.

B. CLINICAL FEATURES
1. Swelling of external hemorrhoids leads to discomfort. Thrombosis causes severe pain.
2. Internal hemorrhoids cause painless, bright red bleeding with bowel movements. Large hemorrhoids can prolapse and cause discomfort that may lead to strangulation and severe pain.

C. DIAGNOSIS. No laboratory studies are necessary. Bleeding is rarely significant enough to produce anemia. If anemia is present, other diagnoses should be considered. The diagnosis is made based on the history and physical examination.

D. TREATMENT
1. **Hemorrhoidal symptoms without significant prolapse** can be treated medically. The use of stool-bulking agents and hydrocortisone suppositories for 1–2 weeks usually alleviates symptoms. If symptoms persist for 4–6 weeks, surgical therapy is recommended.
2. **Thrombosed external hemorrhoids** can be managed as described earlier. If the patient has severe pain or evidence of bleeding or necrosis, local anesthesia and elliptical surgical excision is warranted.
3. **Symptomatic internal hemorrhoids** that are resistant to medical therapy or that cause prolapse can be banded. The band causes necrosis of the hemorrhoid over the next several days. Because internal hemorrhoids are located above the dentate line, they are not sensitive to rubber-band ligation. To reduce discomfort, only one or two hemorrhoids should be banded at one visit.
4. **Fourth-degree prolapse or strangulated internal hemorrhoids** should be treated with **hemorrhoidectomy**. This procedure is performed by placing an absorbable suture at the apex of the hemorrhoid and then excising the tissue. The suture is used to close the remaining defect and obtain hemostasis.

Ⅳ Anal Cancer

A. GENERAL CHARACTERISTICS
1. The anus is divided into the anal margin (distal to the dentate line) and the anal canal (proximal to the dentate line). The dentate line is the area of transition (cloacogenic

zone) between the columnar epithelium of the anal canal and the squamous epithelium of the anal margin. This classification is important because tumors behave differently and have a different metastatic pattern depending on their location relative to the dentate line.

2. Attempts at staging anal carcinoma have not proven effective in predicting prognosis.

3. Tumors are divided into those of the anal margin (squamous cell carcinoma, basal cell carcinoma, and perianal Paget's disease) and those of the anal canal (epidermoid carcinoma, melanoma, and adenocarcinoma). Squamous cell carcinoma, epidermoid carcinoma, and melanoma are the most clinically significant and are considered here. Adenocarcinoma of the anal canal is rare.

B. SQUAMOUS CELL CARCINOMA OF THE ANAL MARGIN

1. **General characteristics**
   a. This type of cancer grows slowly and is usually well differentiated.
   b. Lymphatic spread occurs, usually to the inguinal nodes.
   c. The 5-year survival rate varies with the degree of advancement (35%–80%).

2. **Clinical features**
   a. Patients may have chronic pruritus, pain, or bleeding.
   b. A fistula may develop in association with the mass lesion.
   c. Examination shows a chronic unhealed ulceration below the dentate line. Enlargement of the inguinal nodes indicates metastatic disease. A mass may be noted as well.

3. **Diagnosis** is made by punch biopsy.

4. **Treatment**
   a. If no metastatic disease is present, wide local excision is performed for small lesions.
   b. If examination shows invasion of the underlying sphincter muscles, or the tumor is large, metastases may occur along the perirectal nodes. Therefore, chemoradiation is required. (See Nigro protocol: C4a)
   c. Inguinal lymph node dissection should not be done prophylactically. The procedure has significant morbidity and offers little therapeutic benefit. If the inguinal nodes are suspect, then a radical inguinal lymph node dissection is indicated.

C. EPIDERMOID CANCER OF THE ANAL CANAL

1. **General characteristics**
   a. Epidermoid cancer of the anal canal is subdivided into squamous cell carcinoma of the anal canal, cloacogenic carcinoma, and mucoepidermoid carcinoma of the anal canal. These cancers are often collectively referred to as epidermoid carcinoma of the anal canal because they respond similarly to therapy.
   b. The overall 5-year survival rate is approximately 50%. In patients who have superficial lesions that are smaller than 2 cm, the 5-year survival rate is 60%–80%.

2. **Clinical features**
   a. Tumors located above the dentate line may cause mild discomfort, pruritus, or bleeding.
   b. A mass may be palpable or seen on anoscopy.

3. **Diagnosis**
   a. Biopsy confirms the diagnosis.
   b. Transanal ultrasound may be used to determine the depth of the tumor.
   c. Abdominal computed tomography (CT) scan is used to detect metastatic disease to the liver.
   d. A chest radiograph should be performed to rule out a metastatic pulmonary lesion.

4. Treatment

   a. The preferred modality of therapy is the Nigro protocol (70%–90% response rate), which includes:

      i. **External radiation.** A dose of 30 Gy is administered to the primary tumor, pelvis, and inguinal nodes from days 1–21. Inguinal node radiation carries little morbidity and reduces the risk of late nodal failure.

      ii. **5-Fluorouracil.** A continuous infusion is given for 4 days from days 1–4 and from days 28–31.

      iii. **Mitomycin C** is given on the first day of therapy.

   b. Patients who have residual disease after the **Nigro protocol** should undergo abdominoperineal resection 4–6 weeks after therapy. Inguinal lymph node dissection should not be performed unless nodes are suspect.

   c. Patients who are medically unfit for abdominoperineal resection may benefit from local excision. For small, well-differentiated tumors, the local recurrence rates are similar to those for abdominoperineal resection.

D. MELANOMA OF THE ANAL CANAL

1. General characteristics

   a. Melanoma of the anal canal accounts for 1% of malignant neoplasms of the anal canal. The anal canal is the third most common site affected by melanoma (after the skin and eyes).

   b. Melanoma of the anal canal typically occurs adjacent to the dentate line.

   c. The tumor tends to spread submucosally but rarely invades adjacent organs. Hematogenous spread to the liver and lung occurs early.

   d. The 5-year survival rate is poor (10%).

2. Clinical features

   a. Rectal bleeding is the most prominent symptom.

   b. Most tumors are only lightly pigmented or may not be pigmented at all, giving the appearance of a polyp.

3. Diagnosis

   a. Anoscopy shows the suspicious mass.

   b. A chest radiograph may show metastases.

   c. CT scan of the abdomen is used to assess for liver metastases.

4. Treatment

   a. Tumors are not sensitive to chemoradiation therapy.

   b. Abdominoperineal resection offers a decreased rate of local recurrence compared with local excision. However, abdominoperineal resection does not improve survival rate (i.e., patients die of systemic disease).

   c. Because palliation is the main goal of treatment, abdominoperineal resection should be performed in patients who do not have metastatic disease. This procedure gives the patient the largest amount of time without local recurrence, which can be painful.

   d. Patients who have evidence of metastatic disease may be better served with local excision for palliation. These patients are likely to die of systemic disease before local recurrence occurs.

Chapter 8

Hernias

Introduction

Hernias occur in several locations in the abdominal region. The most commonly recognized hernias considered here are inguinal, femoral, and umbilical. Incisional hernias are defects that arise after surgical violation of the abdominal fascia. Surgical repair of these defects is indicated. Synthetic mesh may be required to create a tension-free repair.

Inguinal Hernia

A. GENERAL CHARACTERISTICS. Inguinal hernias may be direct (i.e., defect in the transversus abdominus aponeurosis and transversalis fascia) or indirect (i.e., protrusion through an opening in the internal ring). Inguinal hernias may be associated with medical conditions that cause increased abdominal pressure (e.g., chronic cough, chronic obstructive pulmonary disease, constipation, left-sided colon cancer).

1. **Indirect hernias** may be the result of a patent processus vaginalis. They originate lateral to the inferior epigastric vessels.

2. **Direct hernias** are caused by a weakness in the transversus abdominus musculature. They are often seen in athletes, and they may be the result of chronically or repeatedly elevated intra-abdominal pressure. Direct hernias originate medial to the inferior epigastric vessels (Figure 8-1).

B. CLINICAL FEATURES

1. Patients have a bulge in the inguinal region that is worsened by the Valsalva maneuver. The bulge tends to disappear when the patient is lying down.

2. Patients may have an irreducible hernia that contains bowel. These patients may have a bowel obstruction and an **incarcerated** hernia. If the incarceration is not corrected, the blood supply to the herniated bowel may be compromised. The result may be a **strangulated** hernia, which is a surgical emergency. A strangulated hernia causes obstructive symptoms and intense pain. Erythema may be evident in the skin overlying the compromised bowel.

3. In men, the hernia is usually easily palpated by placing the index finger into the skin of the scrotum and directing the finger toward the internal ring. At this point, the Valsalva maneuver causes the hernia to protrude, where it is felt against the examiner's finger. In women, a hernia can be detected by palpation directly over the internal inguinal ring on Valsalva maneuver. Differentiation between indirect and direct hernia on physical examination is difficult. This differentiation provides no benefit because the incision for both is the same and the distinction can be made intraoperatively.

C. DIAGNOSIS is based largely on history and physical examination. In patients whose body habitus makes palpation of the hernia difficult, ultrasound or computed tomography (CT) scan may identify bowel in the area of the defect. If a mass is found in the inguinal region,

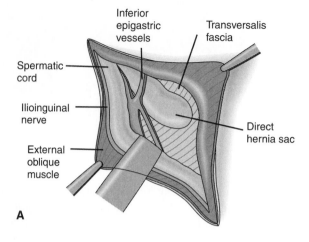

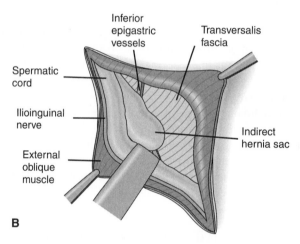

● **Figure 8.1** Inguinal hernias. (*A*) A direct hernia is a defect through the inguinal floor medial to the inferior epigastric vessels. (*B*) An indirect hernia produces a sac through the internal ring along the anteromedial aspect of the spermatic cord, which lies lateral to the inferior epigastric vessels.

CT or ultrasound is useful in differentiating a hernia from other causes (e.g., lipoma, adenopathy, hydrocele, neoplasm).

   D. TREATMENT. Surgery is recommended because an unrepaired hernia may progress to incarceration or strangulation that requires emergent surgical intervention.
   1. A variety of techniques for repair have been used over several decades. The most common type is **synthetic mesh repair.** This technique involves suturing the mesh to the shelving edge of the inguinal ligament, the pubis, and the internal oblique. The tail of the mesh is cut to fit around the spermatic cord as it exits the internal ring. The mesh is sutured snugly superolateral to the internal ring (Figure 8-2).
   2. Other repairs that are less common include:
      a. **Bassini repair.** This technique involves suturing the transversus abdominus and transversalis fascia to the shelving edge of the inguinal ligament after the inguinal floor structures are divided.
      b. **Shouldice repair.** This technique is similar to the Bassini repair, except that the approximation to the inguinal ligament is performed in an overlapping fashion.

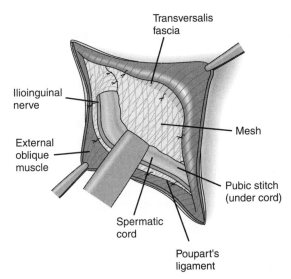

● Figure 8.2 Repair of an inguinal hernia with synthetic mesh. The spermatic cord is reflected laterally, and the mesh is sutured to the pubic tubercle, the transversalis fascia superolaterally, and Poupart's ligament inferolaterally. The mesh is cut to fit around the spermatic cord to secure the internal ring snugly but not to constrict it.

    c.   **McVay repair.** This technique involves excising the attenuated inguinal floor to expose Cooper's ligament. The conjoined tendon structures are approximated to Cooper's ligament.

  3. The hernia sac is dissected from surrounding structures. The sac is highly ligated after it is opened to ensure that it does not contain intra-abdominal contents. An indirect hernia is dissected before the defect is repaired.

  4. If tension occurs with any type of repair, a relaxing incision can be made in the transversalis fascia. The mesh repair creates a tension-free repair without the need for a relaxing incision.

Ⅲ Femoral Hernia

A. GENERAL CHARACTERISTICS
  1. Femoral hernia is much less common than inguinal hernia.
  2. Femoral hernia occurs more often in women, but the most common type of hernia in women is still inguinal.
  3. The hernia sac protrudes through an inlet into the femoral canal medial to the femoral vein.

B. CLINICAL FEATURES
  1. Patients may have pain in the femoral region.
  2. Patients may have signs and symptoms of bowel obstruction if bowel is incarcerated or strangulated.
  3. A bulge may be palpable medial to the femoral pulse and inferior to the inguinal ligament.

C. DIAGNOSIS is usually made by history and physical examination. If physical examination does not show an obvious hernia, CT scan or ultrasound may show protruding bowel inferior to the inguinal ligament adjacent to the femoral vessels.

D. TREATMENT. Surgical repair involves approximating the iliopubic tract to Cooper's ligament medial to the femoral vein, thereby obliterating the femoral canal. Before the defect is closed, the hernia sac is dissected from surrounding structures. After the sac is opened, it is highly ligated to ensure that it contains no intra-abdominal contents.

Ⅳ **Umbilical Hernia**

A. GENERAL CHARACTERISTICS

1. Umbilical hernia results from an abdominal wall defect at the umbilicus.
2. In children, the defect is usually congenital. In adults, most umbilical hernias are acquired and were not present during infancy. Those that occur in adults are typically paraumbilical hernias.
3. Umbilical hernias are more common in multiparous women and in those with conditions that cause chronically increased abdominal pressure (e.g., ascites).

B. CLINICAL FEATURES

1. Patients notice a bulge and often have discomfort that worsens with Valsalva maneuver or straining.
2. Incarceration or strangulation may occur and may cause the signs and symptoms of bowel obstruction.
3. Overlying erythema of the skin suggests underlying bowel necrosis and strangulation when the hernia cannot be reduced.

C. DIAGNOSIS. History and physical examination is usually sufficient, but CT scan or ultrasound may be useful in patients whose hernia is not easily palpable.

D. TREATMENT. Umbilical hernias may spontaneously close in children. Therefore, surgery usually is not undertaken until the hernia defect persists beyond 4 years of age. In adults, the hernia defect should be repaired. When the defect is small and the fascial edges can be reapproximated without significant tension (usually <2–3 cm), simple interrupted suture may be used for the repair. In larger defects, synthetic mesh is used to construct a tension-free repair.

Chapter 9

Disorders of the Pancreas

I. Acute Pancreatitis

A. GENERAL CHARACTERISTICS

1. Acute pancreatitis is a disorder of the exocrine pancreas. It is associated with acinar cell injury, and it causes local and systemic inflammatory responses of varying degrees.
2. Most patients have simple, edematous pancreatitis that is self-limited. Fulminant pancreatic necrosis (which may be irreversible) with multiorgan system failure occurs in 5%–10% of patients.
3. The pathophysiology includes three factors: (1) inappropriate pancreatic protease activation that leads to autodigestion, (2) discharge of acinar cells through the basolateral membrane (antiluminal side) and into the interstitium, and (3) activation of the inflammatory response (local and systemic), with liberation of cytokines.
4. In the United States, acute pancreatitis is most often caused by alcohol abuse (55%) and gallstones (30%). Other causes include recent biliary surgery, recent endoscopic retrograde cholangiopancreatography (ERCP), hyperlipidemia, hyperparathyroidism, drugs, and infection.
5. The passage of gallstones through the ampulla may cause reflux of bile into the pancreatic duct and initiate the events that lead to pancreatitis (common channel theory; Figure 9-1). At presentation, most patients have passed their gallstone through the ampulla.
6. Ethanol leads to pancreatitis by increasing ductal pressures when protein is deposited within the pancreatic duct and ampullary tension increases as a result. Pancreatic enzyme secretion also increases with ethanol ingestion. These two factors enhance the entry of protease into the pancreatic interstitium and cause subsequent inflammation.

B. CLINICAL FEATURES

1. Epigastric pain may be mild to severe and radiates to the back.
2. Patients often have nausea and multiple episodes of emesis.
3. If the condition is severe, hypotension or tachycardia may be present.
4. If hemorrhagic necrosis is present, flank ecchymosis (Grey Turner sign) or periumbilical ecchymosis (Cullen sign) may occur.
5. Any combination of multiorgan system failure, systemic inflammatory response, and acute respiratory distress syndrome may develop.

C. DIAGNOSIS

1. Abdominal radiographs may show a sentinel loop of bowel in the left upper quadrant. This loop is nonspecific for pancreatitis. An associated left-sided pleural effusion may occur as well.
2. Serum amylase and lipase levels are usually elevated. The degree of elevation does not correlate with the intensity of the disease.

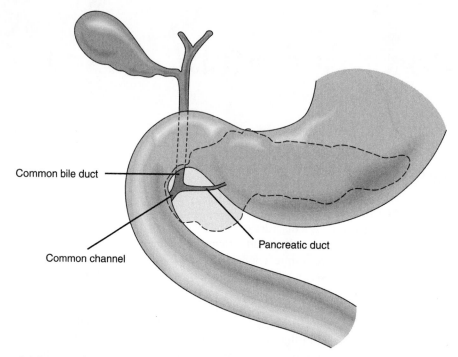

● **Figure 9.1** Common channel theory. The pancreatic duct joins the common bile duct as the two ducts enter the ampulla. The stone passes through the common channel and causes bile reflux. Increased pressure into the pancreatic duct produces pancreatitis.

3. Ultrasound may show an echolucent and enlarged gland. It also provides information about gallstones as an etiologic factor.
4. Computed tomography (CT) scan shows an edematous or necrotic pancreas but is less sensitive than ultrasound in detecting gallstones.
5. ERCP should not be performed during acute pancreatitis because it may exacerbate the inflammation. If the patient has persistent ductal obstruction and worsening pancreatitis, ERCP may be useful in limiting the course of the pancreatitis by removing the obstruction.

D. PROGNOSIS

1. Several scales are used to estimate the risk of mortality. The most widely known is Ranson's criteria. These are divided into the findings that are present on admission and those that develop over the ensuing 48 hours. These findings are as follows:
   a. **Admission criteria**
      i.   Age >55 years
      ii. White blood cell count >16,000/mm³
      iii. Glucose level >200 mg/dL
      iv. Lactate dehydrogenase level >350 IU/L
      v.   Serum glutamate oxaloacetate transaminase level >250 IU/L
   b. **48-hour criteria**
      i.   Hematocrit decrease >10%
      ii. Blood urea nitrogen level increase >5 mg/dL
      iii. Calcium level <8 mg/dL
      iv. Partial pressure of oxygen in arterial blood <60 mm Hg
      v.   Base deficit >4 mEq/L
      vi. Fluid sequestration >6 L

2. If a patient meets three of the criteria, the mortality rate is 30%. If a patient meets four to six criteria, the mortality rate is 40%. If a patient meets more than seven criteria, the mortality rate is nearly 100%.

E. TREATMENT

1. Medical therapy

   a. **Intravenous fluid resuscitation** is usually accomplished initially with lactated Ringer's solution. Patients may be profoundly hypovolemic because of third-space volume loss and vomiting. A central venous or Swan-Ganz catheter may be needed to optimize fluid replacement, especially in patients who have a history of cardiac disease or congestive heart failure. Replenishing the intravascular volume reduces pancreatic ischemia, which may limit the disease course.

   b. **Nasogastric decompression** may reduce gastric emptying of acidic solution into the duodenum and therefore reduce pancreatic stimulation.

   c. **Antacids** (e.g., ranitidine) may be helpful. They may also reduce the incidence of stress-associated gastric ulcer.

   d. Acute respiratory failure is common in severe pancreatitis. **Oxygen** provided through a nasal cannula or face mask may be required. If this is insufficient, intubation may be necessary. Pulmonary function may require support until the acute phase of the illness resolves.

   e. Significant pleural effusion may develop. If it causes symptoms, it should be drained by **thoracentesis**.

   f. **Dialysis** may be necessary if renal failure occurs.

   g. Significant nitrogen loss occurs during the acute phase. Therefore, nutrition is extremely important. Most patients have an ileus and cannot tolerate enteral nutrition. Stimulation of the pancreas can be avoided with jejunal feeding tubes and the use of an elemental formula. In the initial phase, **total parenteral nutrition** is most often used.

   h. Glucose homeostasis is maintained with an **insulin** sliding scale.

   i. **Antibiotics** are reserved for patients who have a pancreatic abscess.

   j. Electrolyte abnormalities are common and must be corrected.

2. Surgical therapy

   a. If the patient has biliary obstruction as a result of choledocholithiasis, **endoscopic sphincterotomy** with stone removal is indicated.

   b. Patients who pass a common bile duct stone that caused pancreatitis should have their **gallbladder removed** after the pancreatitis resolves and before discharge. Removal of the gallbladder is necessary because the risk of recurrent gallstone pancreatitis is 30%–50% within 6 weeks of the initial episode if it is not removed.

   c. Benign obstructions caused by other factors should be corrected surgically. **Pancreaticojejunal diversion** is often needed.

   d. Peritoneal lavage for complicated pancreatitis does not reduce the mortality rate. Therefore, it is no longer widely used.

   e. Patients who have necrotizing pancreatitis may require **debridement**. Patients who have a suspected infectious component should undergo CT-**guided needle aspiration** for culture analysis. If an infection is present, operative debridement with external drainage is necessary.

ⓤ Chronic Pancreatitis

A. GENERAL CHARACTERISTICS

1. Chronic pancreatitis causes progressive fibrosis, exocrine dysfunction, and sometimes endocrine dysfunction of the gland.

2. Chronic alcohol abuse is the most common associated factor (70% of cases). Another 15% of cases are idiopathic.

3. Other associated factors include long-standing hyperparathyroidism, chronic malnutrition, and pancreatic duct obstruction as a result of tumor or stricture.

B. CLINICAL FEATURES

1. Patients often have dull, constant epigastric pain radiating to the back. The pain may be exacerbated by food or alcohol, but it occurs almost daily.

2. Steatorrhea and weight loss may be present.

C. DIAGNOSIS

1. Amylase and lipase levels may be low, normal, or elevated. Therefore, this information does not help in the diagnosis.

2. Pancreatic exocrine function can be tested with the bentiromide test or the exhaled $^{14}CO_2$ test. However, these findings are positive only when there is significant exocrine dysfunction (>90% loss).

3. Glucose intolerance may be present.

4. Plain abdominal radiographs show calcification of the pancreas in 30%–40% of patients. This finding is pathognomonic.

5. Ultrasound may show an atrophic gland with pancreatic ductal dilation. Ultrasound has a sensitivity of approximately 60% and a specificity of as high as 90%.

6. CT is more sensitive than ultrasound.

7. ERCP is the most sensitive test (90%). It shows dilated secondary and tertiary ducts in early disease and a dilated main pancreatic duct in moderate disease. In advanced disease, it shows the classic "chain-of-lakes" appearance. ERCP may also show an anatomic cause.

D. TREATMENT

1. **Abstinence from alcohol** provides moderate pain relief in patients who have alcohol-induced chronic pancreatitis.

2. **Administration of pancreatic enzymes** provides variable relief from pain and may reduce steatorrhea and malabsorption.

3. **Analgesics** are the mainstay of nonoperative therapy.

4. **Endoscopic placement of pancreatic duct stents** provides short-term improvement of symptoms. However, the risk of duct injury and fibrosis is significant, and this mode of therapy is not often used.

5. **Surgical therapy** is most often sought by patients who have intractable pain or narcotic addiction. Before surgery, a CT scan is performed to rule out pancreatic carcinoma. ERCP is performed to evaluate the anatomy of the pancreatic duct. Surgical therapy may require drainage of the pancreatic duct (pancreaticojejunostomy) or pancreatic resection.

    a. Pancreaticojejunostomy (Puestow procedure)

        i. This procedure facilitates drainage of the pancreatic duct. The pain associated with chronic pancreatitis is often caused by elevated pancreatic ductal pressure. If the pressure is relieved, the pain improves.

        ii. The pancreatic duct must be dilated to at least 8 mm for the procedure to be effective and technically possible.

        iii. The duct is opened throughout most of its length and anastomosed to a loop of jejunum (Figure 9-2).

        iv. In approximately 80% of patients, pain symptoms improve significantly. However, malabsorption persists because the ability of the pancreas to generate digestive enzymes remains impaired.

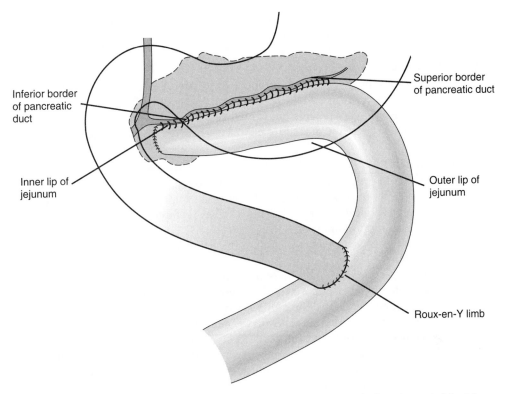

Superior border
of pancreatic duct

Inferior border
of pancreatic
duct

Inner lip of
jejunum

Outer lip of
jejunum

Roux-en-Y limb

● **Figure 9.2** The Puestow procedure creates a side-to-side anastomosis between the lateral aspect of the jejunum and the pancreatic duct. This anastomosis permits the pancreatic duct to drain and relieves pain caused by obstruction of the duct as a result of chronic pancreatitis.

    b. **Pancreatic resection**
       i. Pancreatic resection is used when the pancreatic duct is not significantly dilated.
      ii. Patients whose disease is localized to the distal portion of the pancreas may benefit from this procedure.
     iii. If the disease is localized to the head of the pancreas, a pancreaticoduodenectomy (Whipple procedure) may be beneficial.
     iv. Pancreatic insufficiency is often a problem with resection. Although immediate pain relief is common, many patients report pain at long-term follow-up.

Ⅲ Pancreatic Pseudocyst

  A. GENERAL CHARACTERISTICS. Pseudocysts are a collection of inflammatory fluid (not pus) associated with an episode of acute or chronic pancreatitis. Pseudocysts often resolve spontaneously within 6 weeks in patients who have acute pancreatitis. They tend to persist in patients who have chronic pancreatitis.

  B. CLINICAL FEATURES
    1. This diagnosis should be suspected in patients who have pancreatitis that does not significantly improve within 1 week.
    2. Patients may have continued epigastric pain, vomiting, and anorexia. These symptoms may be caused by pancreatitis or may signal the development of a pseudocyst.

3. Occasionally, hemorrhage into the pseudocyst occurs. This is often fatal in patients who have tachycardia and hypotension.

C. DIAGNOSIS
1. CT scan is the most reliable method used to diagnose a clinically significant pseudo-cyst.
2. ERCP is also very reliable but should be avoided in patients who have acute pancreatitis because the procedure may exacerbate the disease process.

D. TREATMENT
1. If the fluid collection is less than 5 cm and no symptoms are present, a trial of observation after 6 weeks is feasible. However, if symptoms develop, the patient should undergo surgical drainage. Patients who have symptomatic pseudocysts should also undergo surgical drainage.
2. Pseudocysts that involve the tail of the pancreas can be treated by distal pancreatectomy.
3. When pseudocysts are adherent to the posterior wall of the stomach, a cysto-gastrostomy can be performed. If the cyst is located along the body or is not adherent to the stomach, then a Roux-en-Y cystojejunostomy is performed (Figure 9-3).
4. Some studies reported success with CT-guided drainage of pseudocysts. These studies included early pancreatic fluid collections as well as true pseudocysts. Including both of these may have led some to overestimate the success of this modality. This procedure may have increased complication and recurrence rates, and surgical drainage remains the therapy of choice.
5. Antibiotics are not necessary because these collections are not infected. Purulent fluid signals a pancreatic abscess that requires external surgical drainage.
6. Patients who are relatively stable and have a hemorrhagic pancreatic pseudocyst may benefit from angiographic embolization. Patients who are not stable require rapid resuscitation and emergency surgery to control the bleeding.

IV   Exocrine Pancreatic Neoplasms

A. GENERAL CHARACTERISTICS
1. The most common exocrine neoplasm is pancreatic ductal adenocarcinoma, which is considered here. Other types include serous cystadenoma, mucinous cystadenoma, and mucinous cystadenocarcinoma.
2. These neoplasms may be associated with smoking. They are associated with chronic pancreatitis.
3. Exocrine pancreatic neoplasms are more common in men and African Americans.
4. They are rare before 40 years of age and usually occur in the seventh decade.
5. Seventy percent are located in the head, 15% are located in the body, 10% are located in the tail, and 5% are diffuse.
6. Spread to the nodes at the superior pancreatic head as well as to the posterior pancreaticoduodenal nodes is common. Metastatic spread to the liver is common. Invasion of the common bile duct or superior mesenteric vessels is common at diagnosis.

B. CLINICAL FEATURES
1. Weight loss, jaundice, and right upper quadrant and epigastric pain are the most common symptoms. Contrary to classic teaching, the jaundice often is not painless. Jaundice occurs only when biliary obstruction is caused by masses in the head of the pancreas. These masses often cause pain.

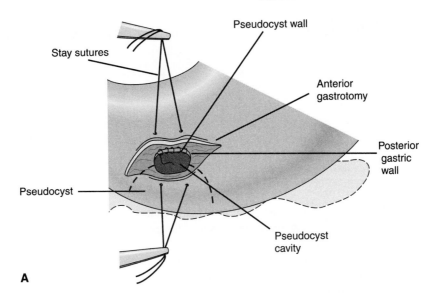

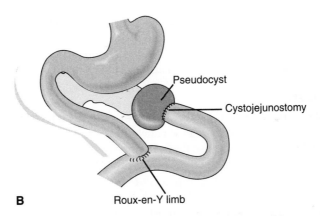

● **Figure 9.3** (*A*) Cystogastrostomy. Gastrotomy in the anterior wall of the stomach yields access to the posterior gastric wall, which is associated with the wall of the pseudocyst directly beneath it. A hole is made through the posterior wall of the stomach and the cyst beneath it. The wall of the cyst and the posterior wall of the stomach are sutured together with a nonabsorbable suture to provide hemostasis and to ensure that the contents of the cyst do not leak between the cyst wall and the stomach posteriorly. (*B*) Cystojejunostomy. When the cyst is not associated with the stomach, a loop of jejunum can be anastomosed to the opened cyst for drainage. The cut loop of jejunum is brought down to form a Roux-en-Y enteroenterostomy.

    2. Anorexia may develop as the disease progresses.
    3. Survival is related to the stage of the disease but is poor overall (Table 9-1).

C. DIAGNOSIS
    1. Levels of conjugated bilirubin and alkaline phosphatase are increased as a result of biliary obstruction by the mass.
    2. Mildly elevated amylase levels (to 300 U/L) may be seen, as are mild elevations in transaminase levels.

Stage	TNM Design	1-Year Survival Rate (%)
I	TI (no extension of tumor beyond pancreas) or T2 (limited extension beyond pancreas, but resectable); no nodes; no metastases	30
II	T3 (extension beyond pancreas not resectable); no nodes; no metastases	15
III	TI–T3 with regional nodal involvement; no metastases	11
IV	TI–T3 ± nodes; distant metastases (e.g., liver)	5

TABLE 9-1   STAGING AND SURVIVAL FOR PANCREATIC ADENOCARCINOMA

3. CA19–9, a serum marker for pancreatic cancer, is elevated in 75% of patients who have exocrine pancreatic neoplasms. This marker is not sufficiently sensitive or specific to be used as a screening test.

4. The c-K-*ras* oncogene mutation is present in 90% of patients. Some centers use this mutation for diagnostic purposes.

5. Ultrasound is a useful first study for patients who have biliary obstruction. Extra-hepatic obstruction without gallstones should alert the physician to the possibility of a pancreatic neoplasm. A pancreatic mass is seen in 60%–70% of cases.

6. CT is often the single most useful test in diagnosing pancreatic malignancy. It easily identifies masses larger than 2 cm and provides some information about resectability. If biliary obstruction is present and a mass cannot be seen on CT scan, ERCP should be used.

7. ERCP has a sensitivity of 90%. It shows displacement of narrowing of the pancreatic ducts.

8. Endoscopic ultrasound is emerging as a more sensitive test than CT in detecting tumors smaller than 2 cm. It is also more sensitive in defining vascular invasion.

D. TREATMENT

1. Surgical resection is the only curative therapy. Most resectable lesions are located at the head of the pancreas. These patients are diagnosed earlier than those with tumors at the body or tail because they present earlier with biliary obstruction.

2. Tumors involving the head are resected with a pancreaticoduodenectomy (**Whipple procedure;** Figure 9-4). This procedure involves resection of the head of the pancreas, the duodenum, the distal common bile duct, and the gastric antrum. A pancreatico-jejunostomy, a choledochojejunostomy, and a gastrojejunostomy are constructed. A feeding jejunostomy is often placed for enteral feeding in the early postoperative phase.

3. Some series from Japan report improved survival rates with extended radical pancreaticoduodenectomy. This procedure includes the Whipple procedure plus:
   a. An extended pancreatic resection to the midbody of the pancreas
   b. Segmental portal vein resection if necessary to obtain a tumor-free margin
   c. Extensive peripancreatic and celiac lymphadenectomy
   d. Resection of retroperitoneal tissue

4. Chemotherapy with 5-fluorouracil (5-FU) and radiation may extend survival and prevent local recurrence in patients who undergo resection (2-year survival rate of 30% versus 11% without chemoradiation).

5. Palliative surgical therapy involves gastrojejunostomy and cholecystojejunostomy to provide biliary and gastric bypass.

6. Palliative chemoradiotherapy improves survival rates in patients with unresectable pancreatic tumors. However, the 1-year survival rate is still poor, and the 5-year survival rate is almost 0%.

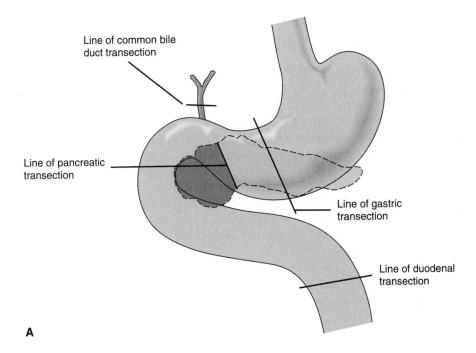

Line of common bile
duct transection

Line of pancreatic
transection

Line of gastric
transection

Line of duodenal
transection

A

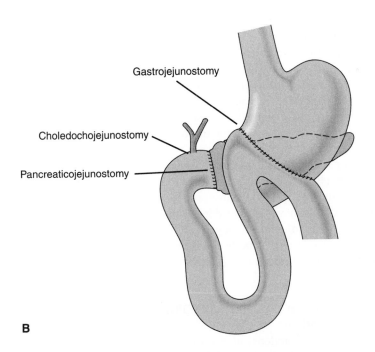

Gastrojejunostomy

Choledochojejunostomy

Pancreaticojejunostomy

B

● **Figure 9.4** Whipple procedure (pancreaticoduodenectomy). (*A*) The *black lines* indicate the points of transection through the stomach (dividing the antrum from the proximal stomach), the head of the pancreas (usually where the superior mesenteric vessels lie), the common bile duct, and the fourth portion of the duodenum. (*B*) Pancreaticojejunostomy, choledochojejunostomy, and gastrojejunostomy are performed.

Endocrine Pancreatic Neoplasms

The five functional endocrine pancreatic neoplasms are (1) insulinoma, (2) gastrinoma, (3) vasoactive intestinal peptidoma, (4) glucagonoma, and (5) somatostatinoma. Insulinoma and gastrinoma are the most common and are considered here.

A. INSULINOMA

1. General characteristics

  a. Insulinoma is the most common **endocrine** neoplasm of the pancreas.

  b. It is characterized by autonomous insulin secretion that produces hypoglycemia.

  c. Approximately 10% of insulinomas occur in conjunction with multiple endocrine neoplasia (MEN) I syndrome (see Chapter 12).

  d. Approximately 10% are malignant, with metastasis to the peripancreatic nodes or the liver.

2. Clinical features

  a. Patients may have the Whipple triad, which consists of (1) symptomatic hypoglycemia during fasting, (2) documented hypoglycemia with a serum glucose level less than 50 mg/dL, and (3) relief of hypoglycemic symptoms after the administration of exogenous glucose.

  b. Hypoglycemia causes confusion, seizure, or even coma.

  c. The catecholamine surge associated with hypoglycemia causes palpitations, trembling, diaphoresis, and tachycardia.

3. Diagnosis

  a. The fasting glucose level is less than 50 mg/dL. The fasting serum insulin level is greater than 25 μU/mL.

  b. C-peptide and proinsulin levels are also elevated. This finding distinguishes surreptitious administration of insulin from endogenous excess insulin production.

  c. CT scan is often the first method of visualization. The tumor may be found anywhere in the pancreas.

  d. Endoscopic ultrasound may detect lesions that are not visualized by CT scan.

4. Treatment

  a. Surgical excision is the usual therapy. Intraoperative ultrasound may be required to localize the tumor and facilitate its excision. Tumors located near the tail are easily removed by distal pancreatectomy. Small tumors located away from the main duct are enucleated. Large tumors in the head may require pancreaticoduodenectomy.

  b. Metastatic lesions should also be excised to reduce the chance of further symptomatic hypoglycemic episodes. These tumors are malignant, but they grow slowly, and patients are expected to survive for several years.

  c. For patients who have unresectable lesions, carbohydrate-rich meals and snacks at bedtime help to reduce hypoglycemic events.

  d. Medications such as diazoxide and octreotide can inhibit insulin secretion.

  e. Malignant insulinoma can also be treated with chemotherapy (e.g., 5-FU, doxorubicin).

B. GASTRINOMA (ZOLLINGER-ELLISON SYNDROME)

1. General characteristics

  a. Recurrent gastroduodenal ulcers are caused by excess production of gastrin from a pancreatic endocrine neoplasm.

  b. Seventy-five percent of gastrinomas occur sporadically; 25% occur in conjunction with MEN I syndrome.

c. Most gastrinomas are located within the gastrinoma triangle (see Chapter 3, Figure 3-7).

d. The liver is the most common site of metastasis.

2. Clinical features

a. Patients may have epigastric burning pain associated with peptic ulcer disease. The pain is typically refractory to medical therapy, and the ulcers may recur.

b. Diarrhea occurs in 50% of cases.

c. Symptoms of gastroesophageal reflux may also be reported.

3. Diagnosis

a. Fasting gastrin levels are greater than 200 pg/mL. Levels greater than 1000 pg/mL are virtually diagnostic of gastrinoma.

b. Basal acid output measurements of the stomach are used when gastrin levels are only moderately elevated. Levels greater than 15 mEq/hr are usually seen in patients without a previous acid-reducing operation. High basal gastric acid output in conjunction with hypergastrinemia strongly suggests gastrinoma.

c. A secretin stimulation test is used to distinguish gastrinoma from G-cell hyperplasia. Basal serum gastrin levels are measured. The patient then receives secretin (2 U/kg), and subsequent serum gastrin levels are measured. An increase in gastrin of more than 200 pg/mL over the baseline value indicates gastrinoma.

d. CT scan often shows the tumor.

e. Endoscopic ultrasound may show tumors that are not visualized by CT.

f. A selective arterial secretin stimulation test may be necessary to localize the portion of the pancreas that contains the tumor if other modalities are not diagnostic. This test involves selective arterial catheterization of the inferior pancreaticoduodenal, splenic, and gastroduodenal arteries. Secretin is injected into each artery, and gastrin levels are measured in the hepatic vein after each injection. The injected artery that produces the greatest increase in gastrin levels is the arterial supply to the tumor. This test is used to localize the segment of the pancreas that contains the mass.

4. Treatment

a. The most effective therapy is omeprazole. Doses of 20–200 mg/d may be required.

b. Surgical therapy is required to remove the gastrinoma and prevent spread. Small tumors can be enucleated. Larger tumors may require a pancreaticoduodenectomy. Careful exploration of the entire abdomen is necessary to ensure that no other foci of tumor are present.

c. If the tumor cannot be localized at exploration, some surgeons perform a blind pancreaticoduodenectomy in hopes of removing the tumor.

d. Patients who have metastatic disease should not undergo surgery. These patients can be treated with omeprazole to prevent ulcerative symptoms. Surgical debulking does not improve survival in patients with unresectable disease.

e. Some studies show a response to chemotherapy (e.g., 5-FU, streptozocin, doxorubicin). However, these studies do not show an increase in survival rates.

f. Patients who are noncompliant with therapy and have metastatic disease can undergo total gastrectomy to prevent the formation of ulcers.

Chapter 10

Disorders of the Liver, Biliary Tree, and Gallbladder

I Biliary Stone Diseases

Biliary stone diseases are divided into cholelithiasis, cholecystitis, and choledocholithiasis.

A. CHOLELITHIASIS

1. **General characteristics**
   a. Gallstones (cholelithiasis) are present in 10%–15% of people younger than 50 years of age. The incidence increases with age. The prevalence is higher in those with diabetes, obesity, a positive family history, or rapid weight loss.
   b. Most gallstones are asymptomatic. Fewer than 30% became symptomatic during a 20-year observation period. Only 1%–2% of patients have significant complications (e.g., gallstone pancreatitis, acute cholecystitis) each year.
   c. Gallstones may be cholesterol (10%), pigmented (15%), or mixed (75%). These stones are typically caused by supersaturation of bile acids with cholesterol. Pigmented stones occur when hepatic infection causes unconjugation of bilirubin and the formation of calcium bilirubinate stones (brown stones). Pigmented stones are also caused by altered bilirubin metabolism associated with hemolytic disorders (black stones).

2. **Clinical features**
   a. With symptomatic gallstones, pain often begins 30–60 minutes after a fatty or fried meal. Pain typically occurs in the epigastrium and right upper quadrant and lasts minutes to hours.
   b. Nausea and vomiting may occur (i.e., biliary colic).
   c. Patients often report dyspepsia, vague abdominal discomfort, and mild nausea after meals. These symptoms are nonspecific and may be caused by other gastrointestinal disorders, although gallstones may be present.
   d. Abdominal examination often shows a tender right upper quadrant. Guarding and percussion tenderness are not usually present. Murphy's sign (abrupt cessation of deep inspiration during deep palpation of the right upper quadrant) is typically absent.

3. **Diagnosis**
   a. **Ultrasonography** is highly accurate. It is the method of choice in the diagnosis of cholelithiasis (Figure 10-1).
   b. Computed tomography (CT) scan is not used to diagnosis cholelithiasis because it often misses small stones.
   c. Liver function test results, bilirubin level, and white blood cell count are normal.

4. **Treatment**
   a. Asymptomatic cholelithiasis is treated nonoperatively, except in patients who have congenital hemolytic anemia and are undergoing splenectomy as well as obese patients who are undergoing weight reduction surgery. Many of these patients experience gallstone-related symptoms.

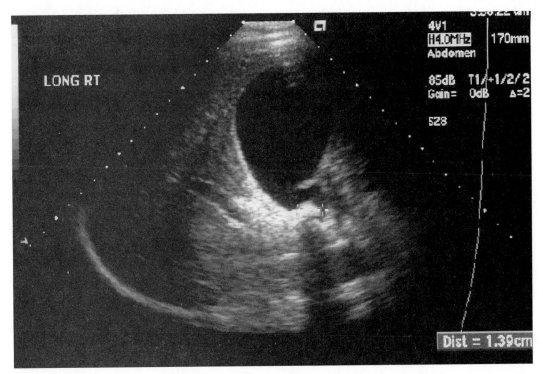

● **Figure 10.1** Ultrasound of the gallbladder shows gallstones that appear as hyperechoic areas within the gallbladder, behind which is the characteristic hypoechoic shadow.

    b.   Patients who have biliary colic are at increased risk for cholecystitis or gallstone pancreatitis. Most surgeons perform cholecystectomy if the patient has had two or more episodes of sustained biliary colic and is at a low operative risk. Laparoscopic cholecystectomy is used instead of an open procedure (Figure 10-2). More than 90% of patients can undergo the procedure laparoscopically. Patients who have intense inflammation (making identification of anatomy difficult), bleeding, or injury to the common bile duct require conversion to the open procedure.

    c.   Medical therapy that attempts to dissolve gallstones with chenodeoxycholic or ursodeoxycholic acid is slow and often unsuccessful. Therefore, this form of therapy is rarely used.

    d.   Similarly, lithotripsy with electrohydraulic shock waves has limited use in patients who have a few small (<3 cm) stones. Complete stone clearance is achieved in only half of patients, and recurrence is common. Therefore, this form of therapy is rarely used.

B. CHOLECYSTITIS
1. General characteristics

    a.   Cholecystitis may be acute or chronic. Chronic cholecystitis is usually caused by recurrent episodes of biliary colic. The diagnosis is primarily histologic rather than clinical. Acute cholecystitis is almost always caused by obstruction of the cystic duct by a gallstone. This obstruction causes distension of the gallbladder, increased wall pressure, and subsequent wall ischemia and can result in necrosis, gangrene, and even perforation with abscess formation.

    b.   Approximately 5% of cases of cholecystitis occur in the absence of cholelithiasis (acalculous cholecystitis). This situation typically occurs in patients who have

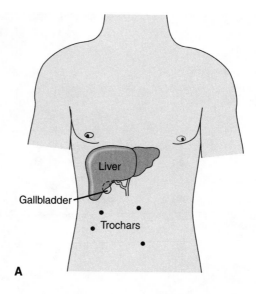

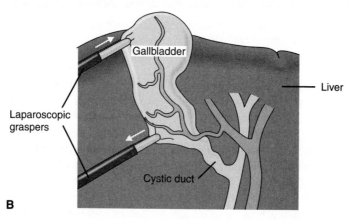

● **Figure 10.2** Laparoscopic cholecystectomy. Note (*A*) the placement of the trocars and (*B*) the positioning of the gall-bladder during dissection of the cystic artery and duct.

generalized sepsis from another etiology, trauma, or prolonged administration of total parenteral nutrition. It is believed to result from biliary stasis and increased bile viscosity within the gallbladder, and it leads to irritation and inflammation of the gallbladder mucosa.

   c. If chronic perforation of the gallbladder occurs, a cholecystenteric fistula (usually with the duodenum) can occur. If a stone passes from the gallbladder, through the fistula, and into the duodenum and becomes lodged in the small bowel, the condition is known as **gallstone ileus**.

2. Clinical features

   a. Most patients have a history of biliary colic.

   b. Patients have moderate to severe epigastric and right upper quadrant pain. The pain is associated with nausea and vomiting that persist for more than several hours.

c.   A low-grade fever may be present.

d.   Murphy's sign (tenderness when the gallbladder is compressed with the probe) is present.

3.   **Diagnosis**

a.   **Ultrasonography** shows cholelithiasis. Thickening of the wall of the gallbladder and the presence of pericholecystic fluid are associated with acute cholecystitis, but their absence does not rule out the diagnosis. Ultrasonographic **Murphy's sign** is very specific for acute cholecystitis.

b.   When the distinction between biliary colic and acute cholecystitis is difficult, a **hepatoiminodiacetic acid scan** is beneficial. This scan is typically used in patients who are at moderate or significant operative risk and who would not undergo an operation for biliary colic but would require cholecystectomy for true acute cholecystitis. The test involves injection of a radionuclide tracer that is taken up by the liver and excreted in the bile. Filling of the gallbladder within 4 hours rules out acute cholecystitis. The test is more than 95% sensitive.

c.   Mild leukocytosis (12,000–15,000 cells/mL) is often present, although its absence does not rule out the diagnosis.

d.   If inflammation is significant, transaminase levels may be elevated. The bilirubin level may be elevated to twice the normal level.

e.   Patients with gallstone ileus have a small bowel obstruction. An **upright abdominal radiograph** shows air–fluid levels within the dilated small bowel as well as portal air. These findings are caused by air passing into the biliary ducts from the fistula.

4.   **Treatment**

a.   Intravenous antibiotics to cover *Escherichia coli, Klebsiella, Proteus, Clostridium,* and *Enterococcus* species are given. Triple antibiotic therapy with ampicillin, gentamicin, and metronidazole is highly effective, but most patients respond to a combination of ampicillin and sulbactam. In patients who are at significant operative risk, antibiotic therapy alone may resolve the symptoms.

b.   Percutaneous CT-guided cholecystostomy is useful in high-risk surgical patients. This technique alleviates the symptoms and infection that occur in conjunction with antibiotics.

c.   Definitive therapy involves laparoscopic versus open cholecystectomy. This procedure should be employed early, within 24–72 hours of the onset of symptoms. Dense inflammation occurs after this period, making laparoscopic dissection more difficult.

C.   CHOLEDOCHOLITHIASIS

1.   **General characteristics**

a.   Choledocholithiasis may be primary calculi, which are stones that form in the common bile duct, or secondary calculi, which are stones that migrate into the common bile duct from the gallbladder.

b.   Common bile duct stones that occur within 2 years of cholecystectomy are believed to be retained stones that were likely present at cholecystectomy. Stones that occur after 2 years are considered recurrent common duct stones. They are believed to form primarily within the common bile duct.

c.   Common bile duct stones encourage the formation of more stones because biliary stasis is increased.

d.   If biliary obstruction occurs, the patient is at risk for cholangitis.

e.   Choledocholithiasis is more common in patients who are older than 50 years of age and have gallstones.

2. **Clinical features**
   a. A patient who has known gallstones and right upper quadrant pain should be evaluated to determine whether the symptoms are caused by biliary colic, acute cholecystitis, or choledocholithiasis.
   b. Nausea and vomiting may occur.
   c. Fever is a nonspecific finding. However, a patient who has biliary symptoms and a temperature higher than 102°F must be considered to have cholangitis. These patients may appear septic and may have tachycardia and hypotension.
   d. If biliary obstruction is present for more than 2–3 days, patients may have jaundice, tea-colored urine, and clay-colored stool. These findings are caused by the lack of bile secretion into the intestinal tract and the accumulation of conjugated bilirubin in the systemic circulation.
   e. Some patients have severe epigastric pain radiating to the back as well as severe vomiting as a result of pancreatitis. Many of these patients have already passed a stone. However, a small percentage of these patients still have a stone lodged in the common bile duct.

3. **Diagnosis**
   a. An elevated bilirubin level greater than 3.0 mg/dL has a positive predictive value of 30%–50% for a common bile duct stone.
   b. An alkaline phosphatase level greater than 110 IU/dL is commonly seen.
   c. Prolonged biliary obstruction may elevate the prothrombin time (PT) because of reduced vitamin K absorption. To avoid excessive bleeding, PT should be checked. If it is abnormal, it should be corrected before any intervention is performed in a patient with biliary obstruction.
   d. Ultrasound rarely identifies a stone in the common bile duct, but it can suggest biliary obstruction depending on the diameter of this duct. A diameter greater than 9 mm suggests biliary obstruction. The acceptable upper limit varies, however, with patient age and previous cholecystectomy, both of which slightly increase common bile duct size.
   e. Intraoperative cholangiogram at laparoscopic cholecystectomy is a sensitive means of identifying common bile duct stones. Similarly, endoscopic retrograde cholangiopancreatography (ERCP) is effective at diagnosing and relieving biliary obstruction from gallstones.

4. **Treatment**
   a. Most patients who have an elevated bilirubin level or a dilated common bile duct at presentation have already passed their common bile duct stone. Repeat laboratory values over 24 hours usually show a decrease to near-normal bilirubin levels. These patients are best served by laparoscopic cholecystectomy with intraoperative cholangiogram to ensure that no common bile duct stone remains. If a stone remains in the common bile duct, the patient can undergo laparoscopic common bile duct exploration or postoperative ERCP with sphincterotomy to drain the stone.
   b. Patients who have multiple stones (>3) or large stones (>1 cm) on intraoperative cholangiogram should undergo open common bile duct exploration if laparoscopic common bile duct exploration is unsuccessful or cannot be performed. These patients are less likely to have their common bile duct stones cleared postoperatively with ERCP because of their size or number.
   c. Patients who have recurrent stones tend to have multiple pigmented stones rather than cholesterol stones. These stones are often large and are not amenable to ERCP. These patients require an open common bile duct exploration with extraction of the stones and T-tube drainage of the common bile duct (Figure 10-3). A T-tube cholangiogram is performed approximately 1 week postoperatively to en-

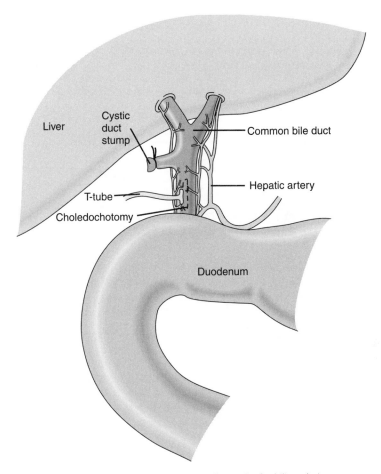

● **Figure 10.3** Common bile duct exploration, with placement of a T-tube for biliary drainage.

sure that no further common bile duct stones are present. The tube can be clamped and removed after 2–6 weeks if normal biliary–enteric drainage occurs. If stones are present, the tube should be allowed to drain as before. A tract forms around the tube over the next 6 weeks. Stones can be extracted percutaneously through the formed tract with interventional radiology.

d.   Patients who have large, multiple stones and grossly dilated ducts are likely to have recurrent stones. These patients are best served by a choledochoduodenostomy after common bile duct exploration and stone extraction. This procedure allows for the passage of subsequent stones and facilitates biliary drainage to reduce the likelihood of large stone formation (Figure 10-4).

Ⅱ Portal Hypertension

A. GENERAL CHARACTERISTICS
1.   **Causes.** Most cases are caused by intrahepatic obstruction to venous flow. Hepatic fibrosis leads to compression of the portal venules. The architectural derangements associated with fibrosis and cirrhosis impair portal venous flow and elevate portal pressure. Alcoholic cirrhosis, schistosomiasis, viral hepatitis, and other liver diseases that result in cirrhosis can cause portal hypertension. Less common causes include hepatic

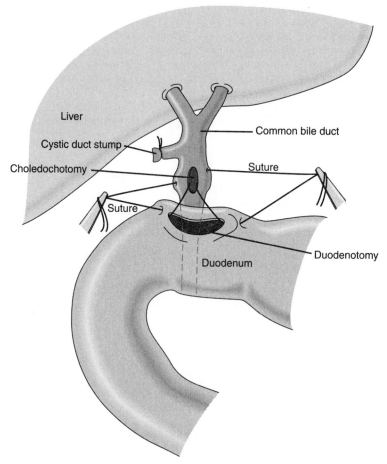

● **Figure 10.4** Choledochoduodenostomy for recurrent large common bile duct stones to facilitate drainage and stone passage.

venous obstruction as a result of hepatic vein phlebitis or venous webs (Budd-Chiari syndrome), congenital malformations, and hepatic arterial–portal venous fistula.

2. Normal portal venous pressure is 5–10 mm Hg. Pressure higher than 12 mm Hg is required to generate varices at the portosystemic collateral sites. These sites include:
    a. The coronary vein to the esophageal veins
    b. The superior hemorrhoidal veins from the inferior mesenteric vein to the inferior and middle hemorrhoidal veins from the hypogastric veins
    c. The umbilical veins to the epigastric veins
    d. The veins of Retzius (retroperitoneal collaterals)
    e. The veins of Sappey (within the gastrohepatic ligament)
3. Surgical intervention is indicated for portal hypertension and liver dysfunction in patients who also have bleeding esophageal varices, ascites, or hypersplenism.

B. CLINICAL FEATURES

1. Patients have a range of symptoms, depending on the etiology and stage of their disease.
2. Upper gastrointestinal bleeding as a result of esophageal varices is common. Patients have coffee-ground or bloody emesis. They may have hypotension and tachycardia if significant bleeding has occurred.

3. A rotund abdomen with a fluid wave indicates ascites.
4. Patients may have prominent cutaneous abdominal veins and caput medusa (prominent periumbilical veins) as a result of reversal of flow.
5. A nodular shrunken liver edge may be palpated.
6. Splenomegaly, which indicates hypersplenism, may be detected on abdominal examination.

C. DIAGNOSIS

1. Anemia may be present if the patient has upper gastrointestinal tract bleeding or gastritis.
2. Thrombocytopenia may occur in association with recent alcohol ingestion or hypersplenism.
3. In up to 80% of patients with portal hypertension, endoscopic examination shows esophageal varices as the cause of upper gastrointestinal hemorrhage.
4. Duplex ultrasonography is used to confirm splenomegaly and identify a dilated portal vein or thrombosis. It also determines the direction and velocity of portal venous flow.
5. Direct measurement of portal pressure with venous catheters is rarely indicated to establish the diagnosis.
6. Significant liver disease may be associated with prolonged PT, elevated bilirubin level, and decreased albumin level.

D. TREATMENT

1. **Esophageal varices**
   a. Resuscitation with intravenous fluids and blood products is provided to restore circulating blood volume and correct coagulopathy.
   b. Endoscopic injection of a sclerosing agent is effective in achieving hemostasis.
   c. Vasopressin (a selective splanchnic vasoconstrictor) is used in some cases to reduce portal pressure and hemorrhage.
   d. Transjugular intrahepatic portosystemic shunts (TIPS) are used to reduce portal pressures to near-normal levels, diminish collateral variceal formation, and control hemorrhage in patients with refractory varices (Figure 10-5).
   e. Emergent surgical portocaval shunts are rarely used but can be if TIPS are unsuccessful. There are several variations, but their indications and usage are beyond the scope of this text.
2. **Hypersplenism** is rarely severe enough to require splenectomy.
3. **Ascites** is usually manageable with medical therapy. For refractory ascites, an abdominal drainage catheter can be tunneled subcutaneously up and into the internal jugular vein to provide continuous drainage (LeVeen shunt). There is a risk of disseminated intravascular coagulopathy when ascitic fluid is introduced into the venous system.

ⓘ Hepatic Infections

Hepatic infections are divided into pyogenic hepatic abscess, amebic liver abscess, and *Echinococcus.*

A. PYOGENIC LIVER ABSCESS

1. **General characteristics**
   a. Pyogenic liver abscesses are the most common type of liver abscess. The most common organisms isolated are *E. coli, Klebsiella, Streptococcus,* and *Bacteroides.* Immunocompromised patients may have fungal or mycobacterial abscesses.
   b. Pyogenic liver abscess may occur as a result of obstructive cholangitis, portal vein bacteremia (pylephlebitis) associated with acute appendicitis or diverticulitis, systemic septicemia, necrosis associated with trauma or malignancy, or direct extension from gangrenous cholecystitis. It may also be idiopathic.

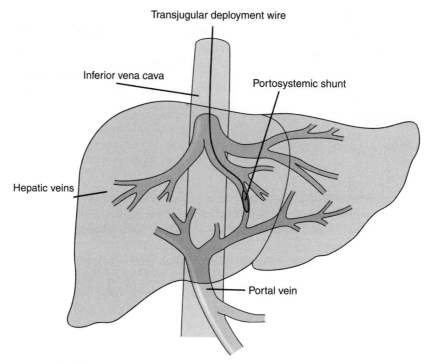

Transjugular deployment wire

Inferior vena cava

Portosystemic shunt

Hepatic veins

Portal vein

● **Figure 10.5** Placement of a transjugular intrahepatic portosystemic shunt. The shunt permits flow from the portal vein to the hepatic veins, thereby reducing portal pressure.

    c.   Approximately half of these abscesses are solitary rather than multiple.

    d.   With aggressive therapy, mortality rates range from 10%–40%.

2. Clinical features

    a.   Patients may have fever, chills, and right upper quadrant pain and tenderness with hepatomegaly.

    b.   Jaundice may occur in patients who have obstructive cholangitis.

    c.   Nausea and vomiting may be present.

    d.   If the infection is the result of pylephlebitis from acute appendicitis or diverticulitis, patients may have a recent history and physical examination consistent with these entities.

3. Diagnosis

    a.   Leukocytosis is often present.

    b.   Results of liver function tests are usually abnormal but are not specific. Elevated bilirubin level suggests obstructive cholangitis.

    c.   Chest radiography may show secondary signs, such as right lower lobe atelectasis, effusion, elevated hemidiaphragm, and extraluminal gas in the right upper quadrant.

    d.   Ultrasound and CT are highly accurate in establishing the diagnosis, but CT may indicate the underlying etiology.

4. Treatment

    a.   Broad-spectrum intravenous antibiotics to cover the above-mentioned organisms should be used. Triple antibiotic therapy with ampicillin, gentamicin, and metronidazole is often successful.

    b.   In addition to antibiotics, percutaneous drainage under CT or ultrasound guidance is mandatory for large hepatic abscesses. Multiple small abscesses that are not amenable to drainage may respond to antibiotics alone. This approach is undertaken only if CT scan does not show a cause that requires surgical intervention.

   c. Surgical drainage is reserved for patients for whom percutaneous drainage is unsuccessful or in whom abscess is the result of a surgically correctable gastrointestinal disease process (e.g., appendicitis, diverticulitis).

B. AMEBIC LIVER ABSCESS

1. General characteristics

   a. Amebic liver abscess is associated with travel to tropical areas (e.g., Central America) that have poor sanitation. Subsequent infection is by *Entamoeba histolytica*.

   b. The cystic form of the organism is transmitted by the fecal–oral route. The organism matures into the trophozoite form in the colon. In most cases, subsequent tissue invasion does not occur. When colonic invasion occurs, the organisms enter the mesenteric veins and lymphatics and eventually rest in the hepatic parenchyma. They cause necrosis and eventually abscess.

   c. The cavity is composed of blood and necrotic hepatic material, creating the characteristic "anchovy paste" appearance. The organism is predominantly isolated from the capsule.

   d. Secondary bacterial infection occurs in 10%–15% of cases.

   e. These abscesses are usually solitary.

2. Clinical features

   a. Patients may have fever, chills, and right upper quadrant pain and tenderness with hepatomegaly. Diarrhea, nausea, and vomiting are often present.

   b. Rupture of the cyst causes widespread peritonitis.

3. Diagnosis

   a. Leukocytosis is usually present.

   b. Liver function test results are often elevated, but hyperbilirubinemia is absent.

   c. Serologic studies for *E. histolytica* are diagnostic and differentiate bacterial abscess from amebic abscess.

   d. Chest radiographs may show right lower lobe atelectasis, effusion, or an elevated right hemidiaphragm.

   e. CT and ultrasound are sensitive means of detecting these abscesses.

4. Treatment

   a. More than 75% of patients respond to metronidazole therapy alone. This therapy should be continued for 4–6 weeks.

   b. CT-guided drainage usually is not required unless symptoms do not respond to metronidazole within 5 days. Patients who do not respond to this treatment often have associated bacterial infection that can be ascertained and treated by aspiration.

   c. Perforation of the abscess suggests secondary bacterial infection. Broad-spectrum antibiotics should be added.

C. *ECHINOCOCCUS*

1. General characteristics. *Echinococcus* is a small tapeworm that is often seen in people who travel in Africa and the Middle East. The tapeworm is contracted from sheep, cattle, or dogs. Once ingested, the eggs hatch in the intestine and enter the portal vein. The resultant hepatic infestation leads to the hydatid cyst.

2. Clinical features

   a. These cysts are usually asymptomatic but may be found after hepatomegaly is noted on physical examination.

b. Occasionally, the cyst causes biliary obstruction that leads to jaundice.

c. Intraperitoneal rupture may occur and cause an anaphylactic reaction. This reaction can be fatal.

3. **Diagnosis**

a. Eosinophilia may be present.

b. If the diagnosis is difficult to establish, serologic testing can be used.

c. CT scan is superior to ultrasound in differentiating hydatid cysts from other hepatic cysts. CT scan more readily identifies the characteristic thickened wall associated with a calcified rim. Daughter cysts are more commonly identified with hydatid cysts.

4. **Treatment**

a. Small, densely calcified cysts are usually dead and require no management. To facilitate resection, deep-seated cysts should be observed until they abut the liver surface.

b. Cystectomy combined with perioperative albendazole (to treat any potentially spilled hydatid material during resection) is curative. During surgery, great care must be taken to avoid cyst rupture. Intraperitoneal rupture can lead to multiple abdominal cysts and anaphylaxis. Before cystectomy, the cyst is aspirated and injected with a scolecoidal solution (e.g., alcohol, sodium hypochlorite) to kill the *Echinococcus*.

c. Occasionally, the cyst communicates with a bile duct. If bile is present within the cavity, the site must be oversewn to prevent bile leak.

d. Some centers use percutaneous cyst aspiration under radiographic guidance. However, the risk of intra-abdominal spill is great, and this therapy is not widely popular.

Ⅳ Choledochal Cysts

A. GENERAL CHARACTERISTICS

1. There are five different types based on the shape and location of the biliary tract cyst. By far the most common is the fusiform (type I), which is discussed here, and starts as a dilation near the origin of the common bile duct extending up to but not involving the bifurcation of the duct.

2. Cholangiocarcinoma develops in 3%–5% of cysts.

B. CLINICAL FEATURES

1. Most present in infancy or childhood.

2. Patients complain of episodic RUQ pain.

3. Jaundice may be present if there is associated biliary obstruction distal to the cyst.

4. If liver dysfunction is present, hepatomegaly and portal hypertension with varices may also be present.

C. DIAGNOSIS

1. Lab studies may reveal elevated conjugated bilirubin if the cyst is causing biliary obstruction.

2. Transaminases may also be elevated as a result of worsening hepatic function from obstruction.

3. Ultrasound shows fusiform dilation of the biliary tract.

4. ERCP provides a useful contrast study to assess the extent of the cyst in order to plan the operation. ERCP may not be feasible in smaller children, in which case a HIDA scan can confirm the ultrasound findings.

5. CT scan may be useful to assess for metastatic disease in cases which malignancy may be suspected

D. TREATMENT
1. Once identified, choledochal cysts must be surgically excised to reduce the effects of obstruction on liver function as well as to reduce the malignant risk.
2. Choledochal cyst removal followed by hepaticojejunostomy is the treatment of choice (Figure 10-6).

Ⓥ Hepatic Neoplasms
Hepatic neoplasms may be benign or malignant. They include hepatic adenoma, focal nodular hyperplasia, hemangioma, hepatocellular carcinoma, and cholangiocarcinoma.

A. HEPATIC ADENOMA
1. **General characteristics**
   a. Hepatic adenoma is a benign tumor that is associated with oral contraceptive use, pregnancy, and glycogen storage diseases. It is most common in women of reproductive age.
   b. Rarely, this tumor undergoes malignant transformation.
   c. The main complication is hemorrhage.

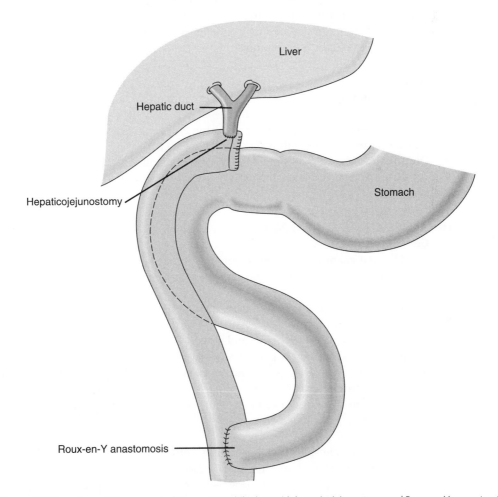

● **Figure 10.6** Resected middle segment of the common bile duct with hepaticojejunostomy and Roux-en-Y reconstruction.

2. **Clinical features**
   a. Right upper quadrant pain is particularly significant if hemorrhage occurs.
   b. A palpable mass is usually found in the right upper quadrant.
3. **Diagnosis.** CT scan or ultrasound is effective in detecting the lesion. Percutaneous biopsy is contraindicated because of the risk of hemorrhage.
4. **Treatment.** Discontinuation of oral contraceptives leads to regression. However, because of the potential for hemorrhage and malignant degeneration, patients should undergo elective resection of these lesions.

B. FOCAL NODULAR HYPERPLASIA
1. **Characteristics.** This benign tumor occurs in women during their reproductive years. It bears an inconsistent relation with oral contraceptive use. It appears to be the result of a hyperplastic response associated with a vascular malformation.
2. **Clinical features.** Patients are usually asymptomatic, and the lesions are usually found at laparotomy performed for another purpose. However, some patients have significant right upper quadrant pain.
3. **Diagnosis.** CT shows a lesion with marked enhancement and subsequent washout of contrast on delayed images. The appearance of a central scar improves the ability to discern this lesion from hepatic adenoma on CT. Gadolinium-enhanced magnetic resonance imaging (MRI) may be used if the diagnosis remains uncertain and appears as a hyperintense heterogeneous mass.
4. **Treatment.** Hemorrhage and malignant degeneration is unusual. Resection is indicated only for significant symptoms.

C. HEMANGIOMA
1. **Characteristics.** Hemangioma is the most common nodule found in the liver. It is more common in women than in men.
2. **Clinical features.** Malignant degeneration and rupture are unusual. Lesions are typically asymptomatic unless they are large (>5 cm).
3. **Diagnosis.** CT scan is accurate in diagnosing the lesion.
4. **Treatment.** Surgical excision is unnecessary unless patients have significant symptoms.

D. HEPATOCELLULAR CARCINOMA
1. **General characteristics**
   a. This malignant tumor is most common among African and Asian men.
   b. Etiologies include aflatoxins from *Aspergillus*, cirrhosis, and viral hepatitis with cirrhosis.
   c. This tumor metastasizes to regional lymph nodes and to the lung.
2. **Clinical features**
   a. Patients may have weight loss and fatigue. Dull, persistent right upper quadrant pain, tenderness, and hepatomegaly may also be present.
   b. In a patient with a known tumor, acute severe right upper quadrant pain suggests rupture of a necrotic area with associated hemorrhage.
   c. Signs of liver disease may be present and may include jaundice, ascites, and other signs of portal hypertension.
3. **Diagnosis**
   a. The alkaline phosphatase level is consistently increased. Bilirubin levels are usually normal unless significant liver disease is present.
   b. The alpha-fetoprotein (AFP) level is increased in 75% of patients. AFP may be used to follow patients to detect recurrence after resection.

c. CT and MRI scans are sensitive means of detecting lesions and planning resection.

4. **Treatment**
   a. The only curative treatment is surgical resection, typically **lobectomy**.
   b. Intraoperative ultrasound is used to delineate the tumor and limit the extent of resection.
   c. Small tumors may be eliminated by **cryoablation** (freezing).
   d. The 5-year survival rate for patients who undergo **liver transplant** is as high as 50% (similar to local resection). This procedure is best suited for patients who cannot tolerate a significant resection because of significant liver disease.

E. CHOLANGIOCARCINOMA

1. **General characteristics**
   a. Cholangiocarcinoma is a malignant tumor that arises from the biliary duct. Most of these tumors are adenocarcinoma. Approximately 40% are located at the common bile duct, 30% are located at the common hepatic duct, and 20% are located at the bifurcation of the left and right hepatic ducts (Klatskin tumor).
   b. Most tumors occur in the sixth decade. Approximately 3000 cases are reported each year.
   c. The etiology is unknown, but patients who have choledochal cysts, sclerosing cholangitis, ulcerative colitis, or clonorchiasis are at increased risk.
   d. These tumors metastasize to the hepatic parenchyma, regional lymph nodes, peritoneal surface, and eventually to the lungs.

2. **Clinical features**
   a. Most patients have jaundice. They may also have pruritus, fatigue, anorexia, and weight loss.
   b. A palpable right upper quadrant mass may be the result of a distended gallbladder caused by biliary obstruction.
   c. Right upper quadrant pain, fever, and tachycardia with sepsis may occur if cholangitis is caused by biliary obstruction.

3. **Diagnosis**
   a. Patients usually have a markedly elevated serum bilirubin level (>10 mg/dL).
   b. Results of alkaline phosphatase and other liver function tests are typically mildly elevated. PT is usually elevated because absorption of vitamin K is impaired. PT should be corrected before any invasive procedures are performed.
   c. Levels of other tumor markers (e.g., AFP, carcinoembryonic antigen) are usually normal, but the CA19–9 level may be elevated.
   d. Ultrasound and CT scan may identify mass lesions and metastatic disease.
   e. ERCP is performed to clarify the anatomy of the biliary duct before surgical resection is undertaken. If ERCP is technically unfeasible, percutaneous transhepatic cholangiogram can be used. Brushings and biopsy can be performed, but false-negative readings can occur. A negative result should not preclude surgical resection.
   f. Once the tumor is diagnosed, duplex ultrasound should be used to determine whether the tumor extends to the portal vein or the hepatic arteries.

4. **Treatment**
   a. If metastatic disease or local invasion precludes resection, palliation can be achieved with percutaneously placed hepatic duct stents.
   b. Resectable tumors are surgically excised. Tumors of the lower third of the common bile duct can be excised. A Whipple procedure is performed to establish continuity (see Chapter 9). Tumors of the middle third are resected, and a

hepaticojejunal anastomosis with Roux-en-Y reconstruction is performed (see Figure 10-6). If the tumor extends to the bifurcation, resection to a negative margin on frozen section should be performed. The right and left hepatic ducts are independently anastomosed to the jejunal limb.

   c. The 5-year survival rate is approximately 20% after resection. Tumors of the lower third have higher survival rates than those of the middle or upper third. Radiation and chemotherapy do not reliably improve survival.

Ⓥ Gallbladder Cancer

A. GENERAL CHARACTERISTICS
1. Gallbladder cancer is most common in women in the sixth decade.
2. There is an increased association with gallstones, especially if stones are larger than 3 cm. However, this risk is less than 1%. A porcelain (heavily calcified) gallbladder has an associated 30%–60% incidence of gallbladder cancer.
3. Most of these tumors are adenocarcinomas, which tend to spread directly to the liver and periportal nodes.

B. CLINICAL FEATURES
1. The patient may have postprandial right upper quadrant pain associated with nausea and vomiting. This pain is similar to biliary colic.
2. Advanced disease is associated with malaise, anorexia, and weight loss.
3. A right upper quadrant mass may be palpable.
4. Jaundice indicates that the tumor extends to the common bile duct, causing biliary obstruction.

C. DIAGNOSIS
1. Results of liver function tests as well as bilirubin level are usually normal. However, hyperbilirubinemia is noted in patients who have biliary obstruction.
2. If the tumor causes cystic duct obstruction that leads to acute cholecystitis, leukocytosis may occur.
3. Ultrasound identifies a mass in the gallbladder that does not move, unlike gallstones.
4. A CT scan should be performed preoperatively to assess the extent of the tumor.
5. Most tumors are found after cholecystectomy is performed for cholelithiasis.

D. TREATMENT
1. When the tumor is limited to the submucosa, a cholecystectomy is adequate treatment. The 5-year survival rate with this procedure is nearly 100%. If gallbladder cancer is suspected preoperatively, the tumor is removed with open cholecystectomy and not laparoscopy. Recurrence at the trochar sites may occur.
2. If the tumor extends beyond the submucosa, wedge resection of 2–3 cm of surrounding liver with portal lymph node dissection is recommended. The 5-year survival rate in these patients is less than 10%.
3. Chemoradiation therapy does not improve survival.

Chapter 11

Disorders of the Spleen

I Introduction

Disorders of the spleen that require splenectomy include hematologic disorders, trauma, and splenic abscess. Tumors and cysts of the spleen are rare.

II Hematologic Disorders

In patients who have hematologic disorders, splenectomy is most commonly performed for symptoms of splenic enlargement (e.g., pain) as well as to reduce sequestration. Splenectomy provides a variable response for several hematologic disorders. Unlike the disorders discussed later, glucose-6-phosphate deficiency is not improved by splenectomy. Patients who have lymphoma, leukemia, or myeloproliferative disorders usually do not require splenectomy unless splenomegaly causes significant symptoms (e.g., pain, early satiety). In most cases, splenectomy is not required to stage Hodgkin's disease because of greater reliance on computed tomography (CT) scans. Patients who undergo splenectomy should receive the pneumococcus vaccine at least 10 days preoperatively because splenectomy increases the risk of infection with encapsulated organisms. If emergent splenectomy is performed, the vaccine should be given in the early postoperative period.

A. **HEREDITARY SPHEROCYTOSIS** is a congenital anemia that is caused by an abnormality of the red blood cell membrane. The abnormal membrane is less deformable and is susceptible to splenic trapping. Patients have hemolytic anemia, jaundice, and gallstones. Peripheral blood smears show spherocytes. Splenectomy is curative in nearly 100% of cases. If gallstones are present, cholecystectomy should be performed at splenectomy. To decrease the significant mortality rate associated with postsplenectomy sepsis in children, splenectomy should be delayed until the patient is older than 8 years of age.

B. **THALASSEMIA** is a defect in hemoglobin synthesis that causes intracellular precipitation and premature destruction of red blood cells. Patients who are heterozygous for the disease (thalassemia minor) may be asymptomatic. Those who are homozygous (thalassemia major) have severe symptoms. Splenectomy is reserved for patients who have symptomatic splenomegaly. Splenectomy may also reduce transfusion requirements, but it is not routinely performed because of the high risk of postsplenectomy infection in this group of patients.

C. **SICKLE CELL ANEMIA** is characterized by abnormal hemoglobin production that results in sickled erythrocytes. Sickle cell crisis may develop when extensive sickling causes vascular occlusion. These patients often have symptoms that simulate acute abdomen. Splenic infarction is common but does not necessitate splenectomy. Patients who have unrelenting splenic pain or who progress to splenic abscess should undergo splenectomy.

D. IDIOPATHIC AUTOIMMUNE HEMOLYTIC ANEMIA. The immune-mediated destruction of red blood cells occurs primarily in the spleen and causes Coombs'-positive hemolytic anemia. Steroids are the initial form of therapy, but if the disease is refractory, splenectomy provides clinical improvement in 80% of patients.

E. IDIOPATHIC THROMBOCYTOPENIC PURPURA is an acquired autoimmune condition that causes destruction of platelets. It is primarily a splenic-mediated process. Thrombocytopenia occurs despite normal or even increased megakaryocyte function. Patients have ecchymoses, purpura, and soft tissue bleeding. Therapy initially involves steroids followed by gamma globulin and occasionally plasmapheresis. Splenectomy is indicated for patients whose platelet count cannot be elevated to higher than 80,000/mL with this regimen. In children, the disease tends to be self-limiting and splenectomy is rarely required. Emergent splenectomy is required for patients who have associated intracranial bleeding. Splenectomy achieves cure in 80% of cases. If the patient has a recurrence after splenectomy, a technetium scan may show an accessory spleen, which may be removed.

F. THROMBOTIC THROMBOCYTOPENIC PURPURA results from the occlusion of small vessels throughout the body. These patients have a pentad of symptoms: (1) purpura, (2) renal failure, (3) hemolytic anemia, (4) fever, and (5) mental status changes. Plasmapheresis usually reverses the process. However, if it is unsuccessful, splenectomy with high-dose steroids can be curative.

Ⅲ Trauma

A. GENERAL CHARACTERISTICS. Blunt or penetrating trauma to the spleen may necessitate its removal because of bleeding. Left-sided rib fractures (nos. 9, 10, and 11) should alert the physician to possible associated splenic injury. Splenic injuries are graded on the basis of CT scan appearance (Table 11-1).

B. CLINICAL FEATURES
1. Left upper quadrant pain and guarding may be present.
2. Patients may have Kehr's sign (i.e., pain in the left shoulder referred from diaphragmatic irritation as a result of perisplenic blood).
3. Significant bleeding may lead to tachycardia and hypotension.

C. DIAGNOSIS
1. Patients who have traumatic injuries with signs of shock and peritonitis must be assumed to have intra-abdominal hemorrhage.
2. The hemoglobin level decreases.

TABLE 11-1	SPLENIC INJURY SCALE
Grade	**Injury**
I	Hematoma <10% or laceration <1 cm
II	Hematoma 10%–50% or laceration 1–3 cm
III	Hematoma >50% or laceration >3 cm
IV	Laceration involving hilar vessels
V	Completely shattered spleen

   3. Ultrasound in the emergency department shows intra-abdominal fluid (blood) around the spleen.
   4. CT scan shows splenic injury but does not indicate the need for operative therapy.

D. TREATMENT
   1. Many patients who have splenic injury do not require splenectomy because their bleeding stops spontaneously. Criteria for **nonoperative management** include:
   a. Hemodynamic stability
   b. Absence of other intra-abdominal injury that requires operation
   c. Absence of active bleeding on CT (blushing of contrast)
   d. Transfusion requirements of less than 2 units for splenic-related blood loss
   2. Emergent intervention is required for patients who are hemodynamically unstable or who require multiple transfusions because of splenic injury. Splenectomy is usually the procedure of choice. **Angioembolization of the splenic artery** successfully stops bleeding in patients who are relatively stable and have slow, continuous blood loss.
   3. The patient with nonoperatively managed splenic injury typically can return to normal activity in 6–8 weeks.

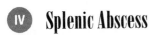 **Splenic Abscess**

A. GENERAL CHARACTERISTICS
   1. Two-thirds of cases are caused by hematogenous spread from endocarditis, pyelonephritis, or intravenous drug abuse.
   2. Other causes are related to infection of a traumatic hematoma, splenic infarction, or spread from perforated adjacent organs (e.g., stomach, colon).
   3. *Staphylococcus* and *Streptococcus* are the most common pathogens. Gram-negative rods and anaerobes are isolated in 15%–30% of cases.

B. CLINICAL FEATURES
   1. Fever and tachycardia
   2. Left upper quadrant tenderness and guarding
   3. Splenomegaly
   4. Kehr's sign

C. DIAGNOSIS
   1. Leukocytosis is possible.
   2. Chest radiograph may show an elevated left hemidiaphragm or pleural effusion.
   3. CT is diagnostic, showing a nonenhancing abscess cavity. Multiple loculations suggest fungal infection. These are more likely to occur in immunocompromised patients.

D. TREATMENT
   1. Broad-spectrum antibiotics are administered.
   2. CT-guided drainage can be used for a well-contained abscess.
   3. Most patients require splenectomy, which is the standard of practice. Preoperative bowel preparation should be considered because significant pericolonic inflammation may be present. In this case, bowel resection is needed to facilitate splenectomy.
   4. Complications of splenectomy include atelectasis, left-sided pleural effusion, pneumonia, subphrenic abscess, pancreatic injury with fistula or pseudocyst, thrombocytosis, and overwhelming postsplenectomy sepsis.

Chapter 12

Breast and Endocrinologic Disorders

I. Benign Thyroid Diseases

Benign thyroid diseases that require surgical intervention include Graves' disease, toxic diffuse goiter, and Hashimoto's thyroiditis.

A. GRAVES' DISEASE

1. **General characteristics.** Graves' disease is the most common cause of hyperthyroidism. It is caused by an autoimmune disorder and results in the production of thyroid-stimulating immunoglobulins. It is more common in women than in men.

2. **Clinical features.** Symptoms associated with hyperthyroidism include heat intolerance, increased appetite, weight loss, sweating, palpitations, and tremor. Older patients may initially have new-onset atrial fibrillation. Common clinical features include:
   a. **Exophthalmos**, characterized by spasm of the upper eyelid, lid retraction, proptosis, and periorbital swelling
   b. **Goiter** (i.e., enlargement of the thyroid gland)

3. **Diagnosis** is made by the following laboratory tests:
   a. Increased triiodothyronine (T_3) and thyroxin (T_4) levels and a decreased thyroid-stimulating hormone (TSH) level
   b. Diffusely increased iodine 131 (I^{131}) uptake in a symmetrically enlarged gland (which differentiates Graves' disease from other causes of hyperthyroidism)

4. **Treatment**
   a. The first line of therapy is usually inhibition of iodine organification with antithyroid drugs (propylthiouracil or methimazole). The usual course of therapy is 6 months.
      i. If the disease recurs after a course of therapy, it is not likely to respond to a second course.
      ii. Patients who are older than 55 years of age and those who have a large goiter or severe, long-standing hyperthyroidism are unlikely to respond to medical therapy.
      iii. Remission rates after medical therapy range from 30%–60%.
      iv. Propranolol may be used to relieve symptoms initially because the efficacy of antithyroid drugs may not become apparent for 2–3 weeks.
   b. Radioiodine ablation may be used if medical therapy is unsuccessful. However, hypothyroidism occurs in as many as 20% of patients who undergo this treatment.
   c. Surgery is indicated when medical therapy fails as well as for patients who have a large goiter or a history of noncompliance.
      i. Patients who have thyrotoxicosis require preoperative stabilization with propranolol.
      ii. Subtotal thyroidectomy (removing nearly all of both lobes) usually achieves euthyroidism. The incidence of recurrence is low.

B. **TOXIC DIFFUSE MULTINODULAR GOITER**
1. **General characteristics.** This type of goiter usually occurs in women older than 50 years of age. These patients often have a multinodular goiter for many years. The goiter insidiously leads to hyperthyroidism.
   a. Unlike Graves' disease, this disorder is caused by autonomous functioning thyroid nodules.
   b. Occasionally, hyperthyroidism is caused by a single toxic nodule.
2. **Clinical features** include:
   a. Symptoms of hyperthyroidism (see I A 2)
   b. Palpable multinodular goiter
   c. Large goiter that causes airway compromise
3. **Diagnosis**
   a. T_3 and T_4 levels are increased.
   b. I^{131} uptake shows focal areas of increased uptake.
   c. Ultrasound shows a multinodular gland.
4. **Treatment.** Surgical therapy is typically the first choice, especially when the airway is compromised. **Subtotal thyroidectomy** alleviates symptoms. Postoperatively, patients are given thyroid replacement therapy to reduce TSH levels and prevent recurrence.

C. **HASHIMOTO'S THYROIDITIS**
1. **General characteristics**
   a. Hashimoto's thyroiditis is a chronic lymphocytic thyroiditis that causes a diffuse goiter. It is most common in middle-aged women.
   b. Hashimoto's thyroiditis is an autoimmune disease. Antithyroglobulin antibodies cause a defect in the normal synthesis of thyroid hormone. This defect increases TSH-mediated thyroid stimulation and leads to the development of a goiter.
   c. These patients have an increased incidence of thyroid carcinoma.
2. **Clinical features** include:
   a. Nodular goiter
   b. Symptoms of hypothyroidism (e.g., weight gain, fatigue, decreased appetite)
3. **Diagnosis**
   a. Elevated TSH level with decreased levels of T_3 and T_4
   b. Increased antimicrosomal antibody titers
4. **Treatment**
   a. Medical therapy with thyroid hormone decreases TSH levels, reduces the size of the goiter, and alleviates the symptoms of hypothyroidism.
   b. A discrete prominent nodule should be evaluated thoroughly because it could be malignant.

Ⅱ **Malignant Thyroid Diseases**
Malignant thyroid diseases include papillary carcinoma, follicular carcinoma, Hürthle cell carcinoma, anaplastic carcinoma, and medullary carcinoma.

A. **PAPILLARY CARCINOMA**
1. **General characteristics**
   a. Papillary carcinoma is subclassified into minimal papillary carcinoma (tumors <1 cm with no grossly involved nodes), intrathyroidal carcinoma (tumors >1 cm but without invasion of the thyroid capsule), and extrathyroidal carcinoma (tumors of any size with invasion of thyroid capsule).

b. Papillary carcinoma is often multicentric.

c. Metastatic cervical nodes are usually present in patients younger than 15 years of age, but they have little effect on prognosis. Capsular invasion is more significant and indicates a poorer prognosis.

d. Papillary carcinoma accounts for more than 70% of thyroid carcinomas.

2. **Clinical features** include:

a. Palpable thyroid mass

b. A history of radiation exposure to the head and neck

3. **Diagnosis.** Fine-needle aspiration (FNA) is a very reliable means of establishing the diagnosis. Malignancy is suspected in any patient who has an enlarging thyroid nodule and a worrisome history (e.g., strong family history, history of head and neck radiation). Even if FNA findings are negative for malignancy, sampling error is always a possibility. A negative FNA finding in a patient who has a highly suspicious lesion should not deter the surgeon from performing a thyroid lobectomy to confirm the diagnosis.

4. **Treatment**

a. **Surgical excision** (Figure 12-1). These tumors are often multicentric. Therefore, a total thyroidectomy should be performed. Patients who have minimal papillary carcinoma can be treated with lobectomy and isthmectomy.

b. Grossly involved nodes should be removed to facilitate postoperative I^{131} ablative therapy.

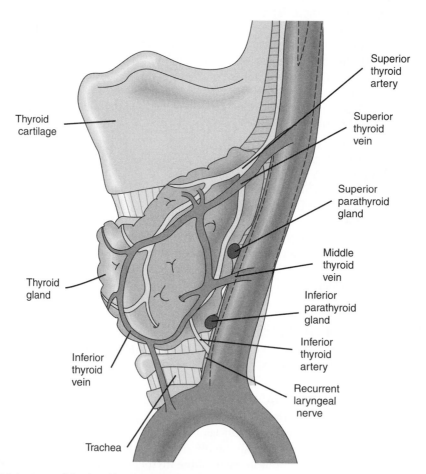

● **Figure 12.1** Anatomy of the thyroid and parathyroid glands.

c. The prognosis is better in men younger than 40 years of age and women younger than 50 years of age.

B. FOLLICULAR CARCINOMA
1. General characteristics
a. Follicular carcinoma is classified as macroinvasive or microinvasive.
b. Follicular carcinoma accounts for 20% of thyroid carcinomas.
c. It is associated with head and neck irradiation or iodine-deficient goiter.
d. It spreads hematogenously and may metastasize to bone. Nodal involvement is unusual.
e. The prognosis is better for patients younger than 40 years of age.
2. **Clinical features** include a palpable thyroid mass.
3. **Diagnosis.** FNA cannot distinguish follicular adenoma from follicular carcinoma. A **tissue sample** is needed to identify capsular or angiolymphatic invasion. Therefore, a nodule that contains follicular cells is considered carcinoma until a lobectomy rules it out definitively.
4. Treatment
a. Generally, **total thyroidectomy** is the procedure of choice. This procedure eliminates the possibility of recurrence and permits ablative therapy if metastasis is present.
b. Well-encapsulated lesions that are smaller than 4 cm may be treated with **lobectomy and isthmectomy.** Tumors larger than 4 cm have a high incidence of microscopic invasion and require total thyroidectomy.

C. HÜRTHLE CELL CARCINOMA
1. General characteristics
a. Hürthle cell carcinoma accounts for fewer than 3% of thyroid carcinomas.
b. Unlike follicular or papillary carcinoma, Hürthle cell carcinoma is radioiodine resistant.
c. These tumors may spread through the lymphatic and hematogenous routes.
2. **Clinical features** include a palpable thyroid mass.
3. **Diagnosis.** Hürthle cells detected by FNA may be benign or malignant. For this reason, lobectomy and isthmectomy must be performed to provide a definitive diagnosis. Permanent sections are required to determine capsular invasion, which differentiates carcinoma from adenoma.
4. **Treatment.** Total thyroidectomy is the treatment of choice because of the risk of hematogenous and lymphatic spread. This tumor is radioiodine resistant and difficult to treat if local recurrence or metastasis occurs.

D. ANAPLASTIC THYROID CARCINOMA
1. General characteristics
a. Anaplastic thyroid carcinoma often arises from long-standing differentiated thyroid carcinoma (follicular or papillary). It also occurs in older patients who have long-standing goiters.
b. It accounts for fewer than 2% of malignant thyroid tumors.
c. Anaplastic thyroid carcinoma is an aggressive tumor with a poor prognosis.
2. **Clinical features** include a palpable thyroid mass or goiter. Airway compromise or stridor may occur.
3. **Diagnosis.** FNA often provides the diagnosis.
4. **Treatment.** Because the prognosis is so poor, even with surgical therapy, surgery is generally palliative to preserve airway patency. In the few instances in which the tumor

is confined to the thyroid gland, cure can be achieved with total thyroidectomy. Tracheostomy with tumor debulking offers palliation to those with airway compromise.

E. MEDULLARY CARCINOMA
  1. General characteristics
  a. Medullary carcinoma accounts for approximately 5% of thyroid carcinomas.
  b. Approximately 20%–30% are familial.
  c. Medullary carcinoma arises from the parafollicular cells (C cells).
  d. The tumor is aggressive, and metastasis to lung, liver, and bones occurs early.
  e. It may be associated with multiple endocrine neoplasia (MEN) II syndrome (i.e., pheochromocytoma, hyperparathyroidism, and medullary thyroid carcinoma).
  2. Clinical features
  a. A thyroid mass or cervical nodes may be palpable.
  b. Signs of pheochromocytoma with catecholamine excess should be sought (e.g., palpitations, hypertension, diaphoresis, flushing) to exclude MEN II.
  3. Diagnosis
  a. FNA shows abnormal parafollicular cells.
  b. Calcitonin levels (from C cells) are elevated.
  c. Urinary vanillylmandelic acid (VMA) and metanephrine should be checked to rule out pheochromocytoma before surgery.
  4. Treatment
  a. **Total thyroidectomy** is necessary because intraglandular spread is common. **Modified radical neck dissection** is required if the lateral nodes are grossly involved.
  b. Follow-up calcitonin levels can be used to identify local recurrence or metastasis.
  c. If pheochromocytoma is detected, it should be resected before any other operation to prevent catecholamine crisis. If hyperparathyroidism is also found as part of MEN II syndrome, the parathyroid glands should be removed at thyroidectomy.
  d. Postoperative ablative radioiodine therapy should be used to destroy any residual thyroid tissue or metastatic disease.

Ⅲ Hyperparathyroidism

Hyperparathyroidism may be (1) primary [autonomous production of parathyroid hormone (PTH) by the parathyroid gland] as a result of parathyroid adenoma, hyperplasia, or carcinoma; (2) secondary (as a result of hypocalcemia-induced stimulation of PTH production, as occurs in renal failure); or (3) tertiary (chronic secondary hyperparathyroidism causing the autonomous production of PTH). Primary hyperparathyroidism is considered here.

A. GENERAL CHARACTERISTICS
  1. Primary hyperparathyroidism is the most common cause of hypercalcemia in non-hospitalized patients.
  2. It usually occurs sporadically but can be familial or part of the MEN syndromes.
  3. This condition is caused by adenoma (85%), hyperplasia (14%), or carcinoma (<1%).

B. CLINICAL FEATURES
  1. Primary hyperparathyroidism is usually asymptomatic. It is detected on routine laboratory testing.
  2. Long-standing hypercalcemia caused by hyperparathyroidism may cause:
  a. Muscle weakness
  b. Anorexia, nausea, and constipation
  c. Renal calculi

d. Bone pain or pathologic fractures

e. Depression, anxiety, and even psychosis

C. DIAGNOSIS

1. The serum PTH level is elevated inappropriately in relation to a simultaneously elevated serum calcium level.

2. Phosphate and bicarbonate levels may be decreased because of PTH-induced renal excretion of these anions.

3. **Sestamibi scanning** uses a radionuclide tracer that is preferentially taken up by parathyroid tissue. This scanning facilitates localization of the overactive glands. Usually, this method is used only when reoperation is required for hyperparathyroidism that persists postoperatively.

D. TREATMENT requires surgery.

1. **Indications** for surgery include:

a. Symptomatic hyperparathyroidism

b. Asymptomatic hypercalcemia, if:

    i.   The serum calcium level is markedly elevated

    ii. Creatinine clearance is decreased

    iii. Bone mass is decreased

2. **Complications** of surgery include postoperative hypocalcemia (e.g., tetany, circumoral numbness) and recurrent nerve injury. These complications occur in approximately 1% of cases.

3. Surgery must be meticulous, with care taken to identify all four glands to determine whether multiple-gland disease is present (see Figure 12-1). All enlarged glands should be excised to reduce the need for reoperation because of persistent postoperative hypercalcemia.

4. If four-gland disease (hyperplasia) is present, then:

a. Three-and-one-half glands can be removed. Half a gland is left to prevent postoperative hypocalcemia.

b. All four glands can be removed. A portion of a gland is reimplanted in the nondominant forearm to facilitate reexcision if hyperplasia develops in the reimplanted gland. This method prevents the need for reexploration of the neck.

c. In either case, some parathyroid tissue should be cryopreserved to permit reimplantation if hypoparathyroidism occurs later.

Ⅳ Tumors of the Adrenal Glands

Tumors of the adrenal glands include functional adrenal cortex tumors, incidentaloma, carcinoma, and pheochromocytoma.

A. FUNCTIONAL ADRENAL CORTEX TUMORS include aldosteronoma, glucocorticoid-producing adrenal adenoma, and androgen-producing adrenal adenoma.

1. **Aldosteronoma**

a. **General characteristics**

    i.   These tumors produce aldosterone and arise from the zona glomerulosa.

    ii. These tumors must be differentiated from bilateral adrenal hyperplasia, which is treated medically.

b. **Clinical features** include:

    i.   Hypertension

    ii. Excess extravascular volume because of increased sodium reabsorption. Patients may have a mild increase in peripheral edema.

c. **Diagnosis**

i. Hypokalemia because of increased sodium and potassium exchange at the kidney as a result of excess levels of aldosterone

ii. Elevated 24-hour urinary excretion of aldosterone (>20 mg/d)

iii. Decreased renin levels in the presence of elevated aldosterone levels, which suggests autonomous aldosterone production

iv. A blunted increase in aldosterone production with postural stimulation, which is more typical in aldosteronoma than in hyperplasia

v. An elevated 18-hydroxycorticosterone level (>100 ng/dL) is typical in aldosteronoma. However, levels are not usually as high in patients with hyperplasia.

vi. A computed tomography (CT) scan that shows a unilateral adrenal mass is diagnostic. However, initially, the tumors may be small and difficult to detect on CT scan.

vii. If these tests do not differentiate adrenal hyperplasia from aldosteronoma, aldosterone levels are measured with venous sampling from both left and right adrenal veins. This sampling shows a markedly elevated aldosterone level unilaterally in patients with aldosteronoma, but near-equal levels in patients with hyperplasia.

d. **Treatment**

i. Spironolactone is first used to inhibit the effects of aldosterone on the kidney, normalize electrolyte levels, and reduce hypertension.

ii. Laparoscopic or open adrenalectomy for aldosteronoma is usually curative (Figure 12-2). Surgical therapy for bilateral hyperplasia is not curative and therefore is not indicated.

2. **Glucocorticoid-producing adrenal adenoma**

a. **General characteristics**

i. This tumor produces glucocorticoid and arises from the zona fasciculata. It results in Cushing's syndrome.

ii. It must be differentiated from tumors that produce adrenocorticotropic hormone (ACTH). These tumors cause hypercortisolemia secondarily (e.g., pituitary tumor, ectopic ACTH-producing tumor).

b. **Clinical features** include:

i. Muscle wasting

ii. Buffalo hump (redistribution of fat to the upper back)

iii. Moon facies

iv. Abdominal striae

v. New-onset diabetes

c. **Diagnosis**

i. Hyperglycemia is caused by an increased ratio of glucocorticoid to insulin.

ii. Urinary-free cortisol and 17-hydroxycorticosteroid levels are elevated.

iii. Elevated serum cortisol levels are detected in 80% of cases.

iv. ACTH levels should be low. Elevated levels suggest a secondary hypercortisolemia.

v. CT scan shows an enlarged adrenal gland. The contralateral side appears normal or atrophied because of lack of stimulation as a result of depressed ACTH levels.

d. **Treatment.** Laparoscopic or open adrenalectomy of the affected gland is curative (Figure 12-2). The remaining gland is suppressed as a result. Therefore, a steroid taper must be administered postoperatively to avoid Addisonian crisis.

3. **Androgen-producing adrenal adenoma**

a. **General characteristics**

i. This tumor produces androgen and arises from the zona reticularis.

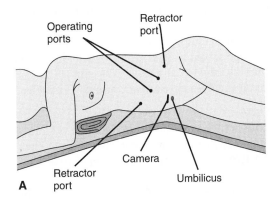

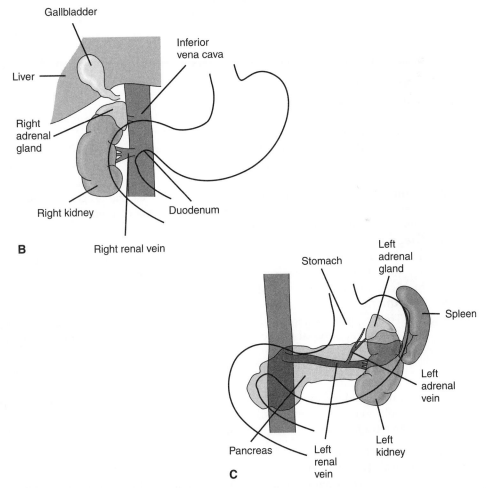

● **Figure 12.2** (*A*) Laparoscopic approach to adrenalectomy and adrenal anatomy. (*B*) The right adrenal vein drains directly into the inferior vena cava, whereas (*C*) the left adrenal vein drains into the left renal vein.

ii.   It may arise from an adenoma but is usually the result of adrenal carcinoma.

  b. **Clinical features** include:

    i.   Precocious puberty in boys

    ii.   Absence of menses and a male hair distribution in women

  c. **Diagnosis**

    i.   Elevated 24-hour urinary 17-ketosteroid levels

    ii.   Elevated serum testosterone and dehydroepiandrosterone levels

    iii.   A unilateral adrenal mass on CT scan

  d. **Treatment** involves laparoscopic or open adrenalectomy.

B. INCIDENTALOMA

1. **General characteristics.** Incidentalomas are nonfunctional adrenal tumors. The risk of malignancy increases with increasing tumor size.

2. **Clinical features.** These tumors are asymptomatic.

3. **Diagnosis**

  a. Functional tumors are ruled out with 24-hour urinary cortisol levels, absence of hypertension and hypokalemia, 24-hour urinary VMA and metanephrine levels, and 24-hour urinary 17-ketosteroid levels.

  b. These tumors are often "incidentally" found on CT scan.

4. **Treatment.** Tumors smaller than 4 cm are reimaged in 6 months and resected if growth is seen. Some authors advocate excision of tumors larger than 4 cm. However, all agree that tumors larger than 6 cm must be excised because of the risk of carcinoma.

C. ADRENAL CARCINOMA

1. **General characteristics**

  a. Adrenal carcinoma often presents late in the disease process as a large retroperitoneal mass (>5 cm).

  b. It usually invades adjacent structures and metastasizes to the liver.

  c. Tumors are not functional or are poorly functional. Therefore, patients do not have functional symptoms.

2. **Clinical features.** Patients may have symptoms of excess androgen, glucocorticoid, or aldosterone production, although this finding is not common. An enlarging perirenal mass with pain is common.

3. **Diagnosis**

  a. CT scan shows a large, invasive adrenal mass. Patients whose tumor invades into the inferior vena cava must be assessed for tumors on the right side.

  b. Screening for functional adrenal tumors is required.

4. **Treatment**

  a. The prognosis is poor, with a 5-year survival rate of 25% if invasion is present. The 5-year survival rate for patients with a locally confined tumor is approximately 40%.

  b. All gross disease, including noncritical invaded structures, should be surgically excised.

  c. Functional tumors are debulked, even if complete resection for cure is not possible, to reduce symptoms.

  d. In advanced disease, symptoms may be reduced with mitotane, an adrenolytic.

D. PHEOCHROMOCYTOMA

1. **General characteristics**

  a. Most pheochromocytomas (90%) arise from the adrenal medulla. The remaining 10% arise from the abdominal paravertebral sympathetic chain.

  b. These patients have an oversecretion of catecholamines.

  c. Malignancy occurs in 10% of patients.

  d. Pheochromocytomas are associated with MEN II syndrome.

2. **Clinical features**
   a. Patients have intermittent palpitations, sweating, and headaches.
   b. Some patients have chronic hypertension that responds poorly to antihypertensives.
3. **Diagnosis**
   a. The finding of elevated urinary levels of VMA, metanephrines, and catecholamines is 98% sensitive.
   b. A CT scan usually identifies the mass.
4. **Treatment** involves surgical excision of the tumor.
   a. Before surgery, adrenergic blockade must be achieved.
   b. Alpha-antagonists (e.g., prazosin) can be used to control blood pressure. Beta-antagonists (e.g., propranolol) can be used to reduce tachycardia.
   c. Postoperative hypotension may occur because of the absence of catecholamines after resection. It is treated with volume and norepinephrine.

 ## Multiple Endocrine Neoplastic (MEN) Syndromes

A. **GENERAL CHARACTERISTICS**
1. These syndromes are a group of endocrinologic disorders/malignancies transmitted in an autosomal dominant fashion.
   a. MEN I consists of parathyroid hyperplasia, pancreatic islet cell tumor, and pituitary adenoma.
   b. MEN IIa consists of parathyroid hyperplasia, medullary thyroid cancer, and pheochromocytoma.
   c. MEN IIb consists of medullary thyroid cancer, pheochromocytoma mucosal neuromas, and a marfanoid appearance.

B. **MEN I**
1. Usually presents in the third or fourth decade of life with hypercalcemia secondary to parathyroid hyperplasia.
   a. Pancreatic islet cell tumor. Most common is gastrinoma followed by insulinoma.
      i. Gastrinoma leads to severe recurrent gastroduodenal ulcers (Zollinger-Ellison syndrome) and is associated with elevated gastrin levels >200 pg/mL. This is confirmed with a secretin test, which causes >200 pg/mL increase in gastrin. Surgical resection to control symptoms and reduce the chance of the tumor spreading, should be considered; however, ulcer symptoms can usually be managed by proton pump inhibitors.
      ii. Insulinomas should be excised because medical therapy for the symptoms of hypoglycemia is limited. These tumors present with dizziness, sweating, and syncope and are confirmed by the presence of severe fasting hypoglycemia.
   b. Pituitary adenoma
      i. Most are prolactin secreting, causing amenorrhea and galactorrhea in the female and hypogonadism in the male.
      ii. May produce bilateral hemianopsia from compression of the optic chiasm.
      iii. Management involves bromocriptine administration, which shrinks most prolactinomas. Pituitary ablation or radiation is used in refractory cases.
   c. Parathyroid hyperplasia—see Hyperparathyroidism.

C. **MEN II**
1. Usually presents in the second or third decade of life with medullary thyroid cancer.
   a. Medullary thyroid cancer—see Malignant Thyroid Diseases.

b. Pheochromocytoma—see Tumors of the Adrenal Glands.

c. When patients are identified as having medullary carcinoma of the thyroid, a screen for pheochromocytoma should be performed, particularly if there is a family history. If a pheochromocytoma is found, it should be removed before the thyroid surgery to reduce anesthetic complications that may occur.

VI Benign and Malignant Disease of the Breast

A. BENIGN BREAST DISEASE

1. Fibroadenoma

a. **General characteristics.** Fibroadenoma is the most common cause of a discrete breast mass in women younger than 30 years of age. It enlarges during pregnancy and involutes after menopause.

b. **Diagnosis.** A fibroadenoma appears as a sharply circumscribed mass on mammogram. On palpation, it feels like a rounded, freely mobile mass.

c. **Treatment.** Observation in women younger than 30 years of age is acceptable. However, in lesions that grow, the diagnosis must be confirmed by biopsy. In women older than 30 years of age, the diagnosis of any solitary mass must be confirmed by biopsy before observation can safely be used.

2. Breast cyst

a. **General characteristics.** A breast cyst is often a tender mass. Most cysts are benign, but in rare cases, a malignant component is found.

b. **Diagnosis** is confirmed by ultrasound, which shows a hypoechoic circumscribed lesion, or by needle aspiration of fluid. The aspiration of bloody fluid or recurrence of the cyst suggests an associated malignancy.

c. **Treatment.** Aspiration is usually therapeutic for benign cysts. Bloody fluid is sent for cytologic evaluation. A negative result does not rule out malignancy because there is a high false-negative rate. The cyst is excised to exclude or treat malignancy if:

i. The fluid is bloody.

ii. A solid component is palpable or seen on ultrasound.

iii. The cyst recurs after aspiration.

3. Fibrocystic disease

a. **General characteristics.** Fibrocystic disease is a normal finding in breast tissue. It is caused by cyclic hormonal stimulation. Patients have bilateral breast pain that may be cyclic, nipple discharge, or breast masses. There is no increased risk of breast cancer with this disease process.

b. **Diagnosis.** Multiple nodules may be palpable, but no single circumscribed dominant mass is present.

c. **Treatment** involves providing reassurance. Nonsteroidal anti-inflammatory drugs or oral contraceptives may be used to relieve pain. Patients who have a dominant mass in the presence of fibrocystic disease should be evaluated for possible malignancy.

4. Other benign breast diseases

a. **Sclerosing adenosis** appears as a mass of microcalcifications on mammography. This mass suggests a malignant process. Wire localization and excision or stereotactic biopsy provides the histologic diagnosis. No further treatment is necessary.

b. **Periductal mastitis** occurs when the mammary ducts are dilated with inspissated secretions. Subareolar duct excision is required for advanced cases, which may lead to abscess formation.

c. **Intraductal papilloma** often causes bloody or serous nipple discharge. These benign tumors are usually smaller than 5 mm. Solitary tumors are not associated with an increased risk of malignancy. However, malignancy occurs in as many as 40% of patients with diffuse tumors. Subareolar ductal excision is therapeutic for solitary lesions. Diffuse lesions may require mastectomy, especially given the high risk of subsequent malignancy.

B. PREMALIGNANT BREAST DISEASE. Two conditions are markers for the development of invasive breast cancer: (1) ductal carcinoma in situ (DCIS) and (2) lobular carcinoma in situ (LCIS). Because they are confined within the basement membrane, these tumors cannot metastasize.

1. **DCIS**
   a. **General characteristics**
      i. DCIS, or intraductal carcinoma, arises from the ductal elements of the breast.
      ii. DCIS is a marker for the possible development of invasive ductal carcinoma.
      iii. DCIS does not automatically indicate that breast cancer will develop. After excision of the lesion and without further therapy, breast cancer never develops in 50% of women.
      iv. Solitary areas or multiple diffuse areas may be present.
      v. The lesion may be high grade (poorly differentiated) or low grade (well differentiated). Comedo necrosis indicates more aggressive disease.
   b. **Clinical features**
      i. DCIS is often detected on screening mammogram.
      ii. Patients who have DCIS may have a palpable mass. Palpable axillary nodes suggest that the mass is invasive cancer. Pure DCIS does not metastasize.
   c. **Diagnosis**
      i. Clustered microcalcifications are visible on mammography (Figure 12-3).
      ii. Biopsy confirms the diagnosis histologically.
   d. **Treatment**
      i. **Lumpectomy** with **radiation therapy** is used to remove the lesion and treat the remaining breast to prevent recurrence. The recurrence rate is approximately 15% and may be in the form of DCIS or invasive ductal carcinoma. This method of therapy requires close follow-up. Lumpectomy must achieve negative margins; otherwise, the risk of recurrence is extremely high.
      ii. Mastectomy is considered when lumpectomy cannot achieve negative margins or does not leave a cosmetically acceptable result. Similarly, if multiple areas of calcification are present in the breast, detecting a cancerous area with mammography is difficult during follow-up. In this case, mastectomy should be considered. Mastectomy is 99% curative if only DCIS is found within the breast.
      iii. Low-grade DCIS lesions that are smaller than 1 cm and do not show comedonecrosis may be treated by excision with 5–10 mm margins without radiation. These lesions have the lowest likelihood of recurrence.

2. **LCIS**
   a. **General characteristics**
      i. LCIS develops in the lobular elements of the breast.
      ii. It carries an equally increased risk of breast cancer in either breast.
      iii. Cancer develops in approximately one-third of patients with LCIS. It may be lobular carcinoma or infiltrating ductal carcinoma.
      iv. Between 30% and 50% of patients who have LCIS in one breast will have a similar lesion in the opposite breast. This finding does not affect management. Therefore, random biopsy should not be performed on the opposite breast in an attempt to find LCIS.
   b. **Clinical features.** These lesions are not readily palpable. LCIS is usually found incidentally during biopsy of another lesion.

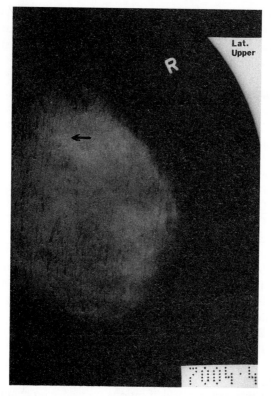

● **Figure 12.3** Mammogram showing a cluster of microcalcifications (*arrow*), representing an area of ductal carcinoma in situ.

   c. **Diagnosis.** LCIS is often difficult to detect on mammogram. Biopsy should be performed on suspicious areas to determine the histologic diagnosis.

   d. **Treatment**

      i. Removal of the LCIS lesion does not decrease the risk of breast cancer in the remaining breast. Therefore, the lesion is not routinely removed other than to obtain a tissue diagnosis.

      ii. Observation with biannual physical examination, monthly self breast examination, and yearly mammography to detect breast cancer early is recommended in this high-risk group.

      iii. Bilateral mastectomy is recommended only for patients who are not willing to undergo follow-up and who desire this therapeutic option.

C. MALIGNANT BREAST DISEASE. The most common malignant breast cancers are invasive ductal carcinoma and invasive lobular carcinoma. The strongest risk factors for malignant breast disease include the presence of the BRCA1 or BRCA2 gene, more than one first-degree relative with premenopausal or bilateral breast cancer, and a history of DCIS or LCIS.

1. Invasive ductal carcinoma

   a. **General characteristics**

      i. Invasive ductal carcinoma is the most common form of breast cancer (70%–80% of cases).

      ii. It occurs in association with DCIS or LCIS.

      iii. There are several histologic variants, including medullary, tubular, and mucinous.

b. **Clinical features**
   i. A palpable mass may be present.
   ii. If the disease is advanced, axillary nodes may be palpable.
   iii. Skin dimpling or nipple retraction may occur with extensive local invasion.
c. **Diagnosis**
   i. Mammography shows microcalcifications similar to those that occur with DCIS.
   ii. Core biopsy or FNA yields the diagnosis. However, even if biopsy findings are nondiagnostic or negative for malignancy, if clinical suspicion of malignancy is high, excisional biopsy should be performed.
d. **Treatment**
   i. Lumpectomy with axillary node dissection and subsequent radiation therapy of the remaining breast tissue is the standard treatment. Lumpectomy must achieve negative margins. Axillary node dissection is performed primarily for staging. Positive nodes indicate the need for subsequent chemotherapy. Radiation therapy to the remaining breast is required in breast conservation therapy to prevent local recurrence.
   ii. To minimize the number of patients requiring axillary lymph node dissection for staging, the use of the sentinel lymph node technique has increased. The breast cancer is injected with radiolabeled tracer and/or blue dye; these substances then travel to the first draining lymph node of the tumor. Using a radiation counter or visualizing the blue dye in the axillary node indicates the need for its removal for pathologic assessment. If the axillary node is negative for malignancy, the patient need not undergo a full axillary lymph node because the likelihood that a tumor has skipped the sentinel lymph node is exceedingly rare.
   iii. Mastectomy with axillary node dissection (modified radical mastectomy) is required for large lesions that are not amenable to lumpectomy. This method is also used for lesions in patients who do not wish to undergo radiation therapy.
   iv. The tumor should undergo testing to determine whether it has estrogen receptors. Their presence determines its sensitivity to tamoxifen. Tamoxifen is generally used after surgical resection in postmenopausal women with breast cancer (Table 12-1). If the tumor is estrogen-receptor–negative, then the standard chemotherapy regimen of cisplatin, methotrexate, and 5-fluorouracil is typically used.
   v. Some surgeons advocate chemotherapy for all tumors larger than 1 cm, even when nodes are negative. The risk of micrometastases increases with increased primary tumor size. In addition, the finding that the axillary lymph nodes are negative may represent a sampling error or a lack of sufficient histologic sensitivity. Table 12-2 shows the prognosis based on stage.

TABLE 12-1	POSTSURGICAL THERAPY FOR PATIENTS WITH INVASIVE BREAST CANCER			
Pathology	Premenopausal ER+	Premenopausal ER−	Postmenopausal ER+	Postmenopausal ER−
<1 cm, no nodes	None	None	None	None
≥1 cm, no nodes	Chemotherapy	Chemotherapy	Tamoxifen	Chemotherapy
Positive nodes	Chemotherapy	Chemotherapy	Tamoxifen	Chemotherapy

ER+: estrogen receptor positive; ER−: estrogen receptor negative.

TABLE 12-2 **STAGING AND PROGNOSIS OF BREAST CANCER**

Stage	Tumor Size	Nodes	Metastasis	5-Year Survival Rate (%)
I	<2 cm	None	None	90
II	<5 cm	Positive ipsilateral axilla	None	75
III	>5 cm or chest wall or skin invasion	Fixed nodes	None	50
IV	Any size	Any degree of nodal involvement	Positive	15

2. **Invasive lobular carcinoma**
   a. **General characteristics**
      i. Invasive lobular carcinoma accounts for approximately 10% of breast cancers.
      ii. The incidence of contralateral breast involvement is increased (3% synchronous lesions; 20% metachronous lesions).
      iii. Invasive lobular carcinoma is associated with LCIS.
   b. **Clinical features**
      i. Invasive lobular carcinoma is infiltrative. Patients have a mass with difficult-to-distinguish borders.
      ii. Extensive local invasion may lead to skin dimpling or nipple retraction.
   c. **Diagnosis**
      i. Mammographic detection is often difficult. These lesions do not typically form microcalcifications.
      ii. Core biopsy or excisional biopsy yields the diagnosis.
   d. **Treatment** is the same as for invasive ductal carcinoma.

Chapter 13

Disorders of the Lung

I Carcinoma of the Lung

A. GENERAL CHARACTERISTICS

1. Lung cancer is the leading cause of cancer-related deaths in both men and women.
2. Lung cancer is divided into small cell and non–small cell lung cancer for staging, therapy, and prognosis.
   a. **Non–small cell lung cancer** comprises 80% of lung cancers. It includes adenocarcinoma, squamous cell carcinoma, and large cell carcinoma.
      i. **Adenocarcinoma** comprises 50% of lung cancers. Lesions typically are located peripherally.
      ii. **Squamous cell carcinoma** comprises 30% of lung cancers. Lesions typically occur centrally and invade the rhonchial cartilage and lymph nodes.
      iii. **Large cell carcinoma.** Lesions arise peripherally and tend to metastasize early.
   b. **Small cell lung cancers** grow more rapidly and have a greater chance of having metastasized at diagnosis.
3. Carcinogens associated with lung cancer include cigarette smoke, arsenic, chromium, radon, and cadmium.
4. These tumors usually metastasize to the liver, adrenal glands, brain, and bone.

B. CLINICAL FEATURES

1. The patient may have a persistent cough associated with hemoptysis.
2. Dyspnea may be present.
3. Pleuritic or constant local chest pain may indicate pleural or chest wall involvement or malignant effusion.
4. Involvement of the recurrent laryngeal nerve causes hoarseness.
5. Tumors of the apex of the lung may involve the eighth cervical nerve, upper thoracic nerves, and sympathetic nerve chain. These tumors may cause arm and shoulder pain as well as Horner's syndrome (i.e., ptosis, meiosis, and ipsilateral anhidrosis). Superior sulcus tumor syndrome (Pancoast tumor) may occur.
6. Tumors may involve or constrict the superior vena cava. As a result, the patient may appear plethoric, with distended upper extremity veins and head and neck edema.
7. Paraneoplastic syndromes are more common in small cell lung cancers. They are caused by elaboration of antidiuretic hormone, adrenocorticotropic hormone, calcitonin, or parathyroid hormone. These syndromes are often accompanied by anorexia or weight loss.

C. DIAGNOSIS

1. **Chest radiography** is the first method of evaluation. A solitary pulmonary nodule is often seen. Calcifications in a pulmonary nodule suggest a benign lesion. A lesion that grows over a period of 6 months–2 years must be evaluated as a possible malignancy.

Hilar lymphadenopathy may be present. Pleural effusion or lobar collapse also may be noted in the case of malignant effusion or bronchial obstruction, respectively.

2. Computed tomography (CT) scan shows the extent of the tumor as well as the presence of mediastinal lymph node involvement. Therefore, this scan is used to determine the resectability for cure. Nodes that are larger than 1 cm suggest malignancy. Mediastinoscopy may be required to assess lymph node involvement before surgical resection for cure. If no suspicious nodes are seen on CT, surgical resection may be performed without mediastinoscopy. The false-negative rate is 5%. CT scan of the liver and adrenal glands is often performed to assess for metastatic disease.

3. **Bronchoscopy and washings or biopsy** yields a histologic diagnosis in more than 80% of cases if the tumor is visible in the bronchial tree. If the tumor is not visible, brushings and washings identify malignant cells in 60% of cases.

4. **Transthoracic CT-guided needle aspiration** is used to provide a histologic diagnosis, but there is a significant false-negative rate. This technique is not routinely used. It is generally reserved for patients who are poor operative candidates when the diagnosis of malignancy is uncertain radiographically.

5. **Positron emission tomography scans** were recently used to differentiate benign from malignant nodules and to identify metastatic disease. The sensitivity of this technique was 80%–95%. Its usefulness in clinical practice is still being investigated.

D. TREATMENT

1. Prognosis and therapy depend on histology (small cell versus non–small cell lung cancer) and staging (Table 13-1).

2. Patients must be evaluated preoperatively to determine their postoperative ability to tolerate lung resection. Many patients have signs and symptoms of chronic obstructive pulmonary disease. This condition can reduce pulmonary function and limit the volume of lung resection that is tolerable. Usually, the forced expiratory volume at 1 second (FEV_1) is the most useful single parameter for predicting the tolerability of resection. A value greater than 2 L/sec is safest for any form of lung resection, including complete pneumonectomy. Carbon dioxide pressure (PCO_2) greater than 50 mm Hg also identifies patients who are not likely to tolerate resection. Bronchodilator therapy is given preoperatively to improve function and reduce the risk of postoperative atelectasis or pneumonia.

3. **Surgical resection** is indicated for patients who have stage I, II, or IIIa disease. Complete resection of the tumor and involved nodes along with involved adjacent structures must be achieved.

TABLE 13-1	STAGING FOR LUNG CANCER		
Stage	**Tumor Size**	**Nodal Involvement**	**Metastasis**
I	Limited to visceral pleura and 2 cm distal to carina	None	None
II	Limited to visceral pleura and 2 cm distal to carina	Peribronchial or hilar nodes	None
IIIa	Chest wall, diaphragm, mediastinal involvement, or extension within 2 cm of carina	Ipsilateral mediastinal or subcarinal nodes	None
IIIb	Invasion of great vessels, trachea, or esophagus, or ipsilateral malignant effusion	Contralateral mediastinal nodes	None
IV	Any size	Any degree	Present

a. **Stage I.** Lobectomy is indicated for centrally located tumors. Although a wedge resection can be performed for peripheral lesions, the local recurrence rate is higher (20% vs 5%). In most cases, there is little difference in postoperative pulmonary function between wedge resection and lobectomy. Therefore, lobectomy is the most logical choice. Hilar and mediastinal nodes should be resected to confirm staging. The 5-year survival rate is 70%–85%. No chemotherapy or radiation therapy is indicated.

b. **Stage II.** Lobectomy with en bloc resection of the hilar, interlobar, lobar, and segmental nodes is indicated. Mediastinal lymph nodes should be assessed to confirm staging before pulmonary resection. Positive contralateral nodes are a contraindication to pulmonary resection. The 5-year survival rate is 40%–50%. More than 50% of patients have a recurrence. This rate may be reduced by radiation therapy. However, postoperative radiation therapy does not increase overall survival rates.

c. **Stage IIIa.** Patients whose tumors invade the chest wall or who have ipsilateral or subcarinal mediastinal nodal involvement have a 5-year survival rate of 20%–30%. Postoperative radiation therapy does not improve survival but can reduce local recurrence.

4. **Chemotherapy** (e.g., cyclophosphamide, doxorubicin, cisplatin) may improve disease-free survival in patients who have stage II or III disease. Chemotherapy is of little value in stage I disease.

5. **Radiation therapy** can reduce local recurrence rates and may alleviate symptoms in patients who have unresectable disease.

6. Unlike non–small cell lung cancer (see earlier discussion), small cell lung cancer usually is not amenable to surgery. These patients usually have metastasis at diagnosis. If the diagnosis is made preoperatively, surgical resectability is usually indicated only in patients who have stage I or II disease. An extensive metastatic workup, including abdominal, chest, and brain CT scan as well as a bone scan, should be done before surgical consideration. Chemoradiation therapy is the treatment of choice, but the overall 5-year survival rate is only 20%–30%.

Ⅱ Bronchial Adenoma

A. GENERAL CHARACTERISTICS

1. Bronchial adenomas are less aggressive tumors that have a better prognosis than bronchogenic carcinomas. The term adenoma is a misnomer because these tumors are malignant. They constitute only 1% of lung neoplasms.

2. There are three histologic types: bronchial carcinoid tumors, adenoid cystic carcinoma, and mucoepidermoid carcinoma.

3. Bronchial carcinoids are members of the amine precursor uptake and decarboxylation (APUD) family. They may secrete active peptides (e.g., bradykinin, serotonin). They tend to arise from the main airways, but they also occur peripherally. Adenoid cystic carcinomas arise from the submucosal glands of the trachea or main bronchi. Mucoepidermoid carcinomas also arise in the submucosa of the trachea or main bronchi.

B. CLINICAL FEATURES

1. Patients with centrally located tumors typically have cough or hemoptysis. Peripheral lesions are usually asymptomatic.

2. Pneumonia may recur because of bronchial obstruction.

C. DIAGNOSIS

1. **Chest radiography** shows a nodule or mass lesion, either centrally or peripherally. Pneumonia or atelectasis may be present if the lesion is obstructive.
2. **CT scan** can be used to assess for lymphatic spread and local tumor extent.
3. Tissue diagnosis is often obtained by **bronchoscopy** because most of these tumors are centrally located and involve the airways.

D. TREATMENT

1. Most tumors respond well to **surgical removal** if negative margins are achieved. Central tumors may require sleeve resection of the involved bronchus. With complete resection, 5-year survival rates approach 90%.
2. **Radiation therapy** can be used preoperatively to decrease the likelihood of positive margins and local recurrence.

Ⅲ Surgical Thoracic Infection

A. LUNG ABSCESS

1. **General characteristics**
    a. Lung abscess is most commonly associated with aspiration, typically in a patient with altered mental status.
    b. Anaerobes are the most common pathogen.
    c. The most dependent portions of the lung are often involved. These include the superior and posterior segments of the lower lobe.
    d. Fungal or polymicrobial infection may occur in immunocompromised patients.
2. **Clinical features** include:
    a. Purulent cough
    b. Fever that may progress to sepsis with hypotension and tachycardia
    c. If the abscess cannot drain through the bronchial tree, progressive sepsis that results in pyopneumothorax
3. **Diagnosis**
    a. Leukocytosis may be present.
    b. **Sputum cultures** often show *Bacteroides, Peptostreptococcus, Staphylococcus aureus, Pseudomonas,* or *Klebsiella.* In immunocompromised patients, *Aspergillus* may be isolated.
    c. **Chest radiography** initially shows an area of consolidation. Once bronchial drainage occurs, an air–fluid level may be present (Figure 13-1).
4. **Treatment**
    a. Initial **drug therapy** with penicillin or clindamycin is most effective. If *Aspergillus* is isolated, amphotericin is indicated.
    b. **Postural drainage and pulmonary physiotherapy** facilitates drainage of the cavity.
    c. **Bronchoscopy** is performed to ensure that extrinsic pathology or obstruction from a foreign body is the cause of inadequate drainage.
    d. Fewer than 10% of patients have indications for **operative intervention** (i.e., abscess larger than 6 cm, bronchopleural fistula, persistent sepsis, and empyema). Surgical resection should be considered if a patient remains stable on antibiotic therapy but has a chronic abscess for longer than 6 weeks. Surgical therapy is directed toward external drainage of the infected cavity. In patients with chronic abscess, the infected segment should be resected.

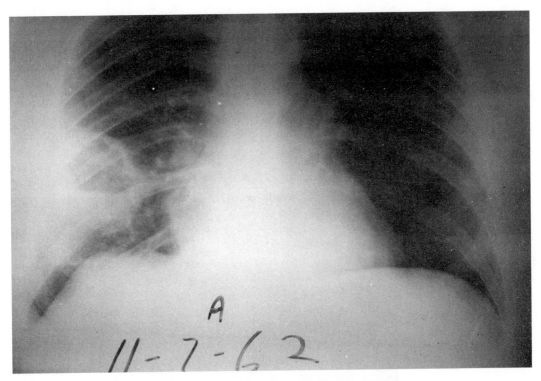

● **Figure 13.1** Chest radiograph of a patient with a lung abscess showing an air–fluid level.

B. TUBERCULOSIS (TB)

1. General characteristics

a. TB is most often caused by *Mycobacterium tuberculosis,* an aerobic, slow-growing bacillus.

b. It is spread by inhalation of droplet nuclei. The result is necrotizing pneumonia that spreads to the hilar nodes. The pneumonia develops into areas of granuloma formation and caseous (cheese-like) necrosis. Initially, the lower lobes are involved in the first exposure. After hematogenous spread occurs, the characteristic appearance of apical involvement is seen. Other areas (e.g., kidneys, long bones, brain) also may be affected.

c. Empyema may occur when lymphatic spread to the pleura occurs.

d. TB is more common in immunocompromised individuals.

2. Clinical features include:

a. Persistent cough with or without hemoptysis

b. Easy fatigability

c. Chest pain

d. Fever and night sweats

3. Diagnosis

a. Subcutaneous injection of tuberculin causes induration in 48–72 hours in those previously infected with the organism. Patients who have a depressed delayed-hypersensitivity reaction may have a false-negative result.

b. Acid-fast staining organisms on smear provide a rapid means of diagnosis. However, the organism may not be prominent. Culture of the organism typically takes 3–6 weeks.

c. Chest radiography shows apical infiltrates and cavitation (Figure 13-2).

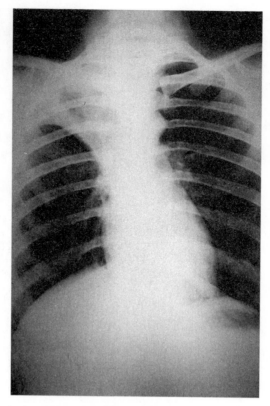

● **Figure 13.2** Chest radiograph of a patient with tuberculosis showing the characteristic apical infiltrates.

4. Treatment

a. Most patients are treated adequately with chemotherapeutic agents (e.g., a 6-month regimen of isoniazid, rifampin, and pyrazinamide).

b. Patients who have resistant *Mycobacterium* infection are referred for surgery. Resection of the involved segment is the procedure of choice.

c. Rarely, massive hemoptysis occurs as a result of hemorrhage into a cavitary lesion. This is another indication for surgical intervention.

d. If a bronchopleural fistula develops, creating pneumothorax and empyema, it may be treated with a chest tube. This treatment usually does not reexpand the lung, however, because the visceral pleura react intensely to the infection. This reaction prevents reexpansion of the lung, and decortication is necessary. If this procedure cannot be performed because of the severity of the reaction, open pleural drainage with an Eloesser flap can be performed (Figure 13-3).

e. Active, diffuse endobronchial disease seen on bronchoscopy is usually a contra-indication to pulmonary resection because it interferes with healing of the bronchial stump. Therefore, chemotherapy is administered to clear the bronchi of disease before surgical intervention is possible.

C. EMPYEMA

1. General characteristics

a. Empyema is the accumulation of pus in the pleural space.

b. Empyema develops in three phases:

    i. During the **acute phase**, sterile inflammatory pleural fluid forms. This phase is characterized by low viscosity, a low white blood cell count, and normal pH and glucose levels. The visceral and parietal pleura are separated.

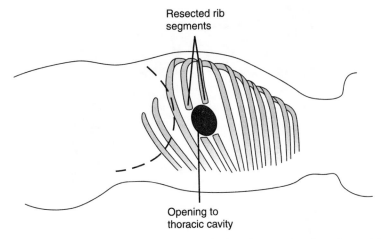

Resected rib segments

Opening to thoracic cavity

● **Figure 13.3** The Eloesser flap, which is created for patients who have intense pleural reaction and chronic drainage.

    ii. During the **transitional phase**, the fluid becomes more turbid, with an increasing number of white cells. Fluid pH and glucose fall, and the level of lactate dehydrogenase (LDH) increases. A fibrinous peel develops on the pleural surfaces and limits expansion.

    iii. The **chronic phase** is characterized by ingrowth of capillaries and fibroblasts into the peel. The fluid is largely composed of sediment. At this point, empyema typically has been present for 4–6 weeks.

  c. Empyema is caused by pneumonia (50%), postoperative thoracic infection (25%), or subphrenic abscess extension (10%).

  d. Gram-negative organisms are often found, including *Pseudomonas, Klebsiella,* and *Escherichia coli. Staphylococcus* is also a common cause, especially in children.

2. **Clinical features** include:

  a. Pleuritic chest pain

  b. Fever

  c. Purulent cough

  d. Decreased breath sounds and dullness to percussion on the affected side

3. **Diagnosis**

  a. **Chest radiography** shows an effusion. Infiltrate and air–fluid levels may be present (Figure 13-4).

  b. **Thoracentesis** is most valuable in differentiating simple effusion from empyema. The fluid should be sent for gram stain, pH, culture and sensitivity, glucose, LDH, and protein. **Established empyema** is fluid that has a pH of less than 7, glucose of less than 40 mg/dL, and LDH of greater than 1000 IU/dL.

  c. **CT scan and ultrasound** are useful in identifying loculations and determining the feasibility of tube drainage versus thoracentesis.

4. **Treatment**

  a. Thin, watery pleural fluid associated with pneumonia (acute-phase empyema) is treated with evacuation by **thoracentesis** and appropriate **antibiotics.**

  b. If the fluid has characteristics of **progressing empyema** (pH <7, glucose <40 mg/dL, LDH >1000 IU/dL), **chest tube thoracostomy** is indicated. If the lung remains trapped because of a fibrous peel despite drainage, **decortication** is performed.

  c. Occasionally, in immunocompromised patients or those who have continuing purulent drainage despite chest tube thoracostomy and antibiotics, an **open**

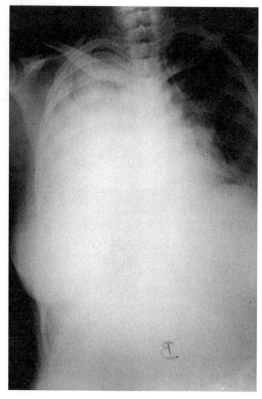

● Figure 13.4 Chest radiograph of a patient with empyema showing an effusion with associated infiltrate indicating a parapneumonic effusion.

drainage procedure is performed with partial resection of a rib over the most dependent portion of the effusion.

 Bronchiectasis

A. GENERAL CHARACTERISTICS

  1. Bronchiectasis is loss of the normal structural integrity of the bronchi. This condition may be congenital but is usually acquired.

  2. Bronchial injury may be caused by infection or by an obstructive process from mucous plugging, hilar lymphadenopathy, or tumor.

  3. Infectious causes include adenovirus, whooping cough, pertussis, *Staphylococcus*, and tuberculosis. Patients who have recurrent pulmonary infection (e.g., AIDS, cystic fibrosis) are at particular risk.

B. CLINICAL FEATURES

  1. Patients have a persistent cough with purulent sputum.

  2. As many as 50% of patients have hemoptysis.

  3. Clubbing may be present.

  4. Rales may be auscultated over the involved lung fields.

C. DIAGNOSIS

  1. Chest radiography may show areas of atelectasis or cystic spaces.

2. **CT scan** is the diagnostic modality of choice. It shows dilated bronchi that extend into the parenchyma.
3. **Bronchoscopy** may identify bronchial obstruction and clear mucous plugs.

D. TREATMENT

1. Conservative therapy with appropriate **antibiotics and chest physiotherapy** is usually adequate for acute exacerbations.
2. **Surgical therapy** is reserved for patients who do not respond to prolonged medical therapy. Involved segments are removed with segmentectomy or lobectomy.

Ⓥ Spontaneous Pneumothorax and Hemothorax

A. SPONTANEOUS PNEUMOTHORAX

1. **General characteristics**
   a. Pneumothorax is the accumulation of air in the pleural space without an apparent antecedent incident.
   b. It typically occurs in young men.
   c. It is usually caused by rupture of a subpleural cyst, bleb, or bulla.
2. **Clinical features**
   a. Patients who have a small pneumothorax may be asymptomatic.
   b. Severe dyspnea and chest pain may occur. If tension pneumothorax occurs, patients progress to hemodynamic instability with hypotension, tracheal deviation away from the side of the pneumothorax, and distended neck veins.
   c. Breath sounds may be absent on the affected side.
   d. Significant hypoxia and tachypnea may occur.
3. **Diagnosis.** Chest radiography is diagnostic and shows absent lung markings with collapse of the lung (Figure 13-5).
4. **Treatment**
   a. A small pneumothorax (5%–20%) may be seen in a stable patient who has minimal symptoms.
   b. **Supplemental oxygen** hastens reabsorption of the pneumothorax by providing air that contains a low partial pressure of nitrogen. This provides a concentration gradient. Nitrogen from the pneumothorax travels over it to the inhaled air and is then exhaled.
   c. Patients who are symptomatic and have a larger pneumothorax are treated with a **chest tube.** This tube usually expands the lung. It is kept in place for at least 48 hours to allow adherence of the parietal and visceral pleura.
   d. If a leak persists, a spontaneous pneumothorax recurs, or an obvious bleb or bullous lesion in the collapsed lung is identified, surgery is indicated. **Video-assisted thoracotomy** is often used, with stapling or suturing of the bullae. **Pleurodesis** is then performed, typically with talc or quinacrine. This procedure causes the visceral and parietal pleura to adhere and thereby prevents recurrence.
   e. In patients with tension pneumothorax, immediate decompression with a **14-gauge angiocatheter** in the midclavicular line at the second intercostal space is life-saving. This procedure is rapidly followed by placement of a chest tube on the affected side.

B. HEMOTHORAX

1. **General characteristics**
   a. Blood may accumulate in the thorax as a result of trauma, pulmonary infarction, or neoplasm.

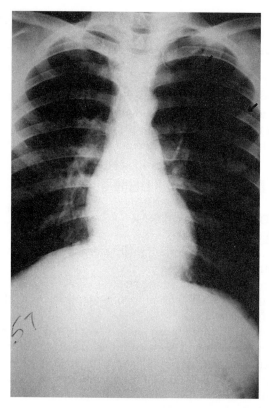

● **Figure 13.5** Chest radiograph of a patient with a pneumothorax. Note the absence of lung markings at the edge of the thoracic cavity. A faint line created by the separation of the visceral pleura from the parietal pleura is seen.

    b. The condition may progress to fibrothorax with lung trapping if the clot is not evacuated or reabsorbed.

    c. The hemothorax can become infected. It is usually associated with underlying lung parenchymal damage from a gunshot wound rather than a stab wound.

2. Clinical features

    a. Patients report dyspnea and pleuritic chest pain.

    b. Patients who have thoracic trauma show a site of penetration. Those who have blunt trauma may show an area of bruising or deformity.

    c. Breath sounds may be reduced on the affected side if significant hemothorax is present. Significant hemorrhage may cause hypotension and tachycardia.

    d. Patients with associated tension pneumothorax may have tracheal deviation and distended neck veins with hypotension.

    e. Subcutaneous air (subcutaneous emphyema) may be palpated over the affected hemothorax.

3. Diagnosis

    a. In the emergency setting, when a patient is unstable with signs of tension pneumothorax or obvious chest trauma and respiratory compromise, confirmation with a chest radiograph is not necessary. Immediate decompression with an angiocatheter (described above) is indicated, with subsequent chest tube placement.

    b. In a relatively stable patient, a supine chest radiograph shows a haze over the entire affected lung field. An upright film shows an effusion that blunts the costophrenic angle.

4. Treatment
a. Unstable patients who have suspected hemothorax should undergo prompt angiocatheter decompression followed by tube thoracostomy.
b. In many cases, a traumatic hemothorax stops bleeding spontaneously. However, if ongoing blood loss occurs, or if the patient remains unstable despite transfusion and tube thoracostomy drainage, then the patient should undergo thoracotomy to achieve definitive control of the hemorrhagic site. Typically, hemorrhagic chest tube output of more than 200–300 mL/hr for 4 hours is an indication for thoracotomy, even if the patient is stable. This amount of bleeding indicates an injury that is not likely to clot spontaneously.
c. When a tube thoracostomy is performed and the patient spontaneously stops hemorrhaging, a subsequent chest radiograph may show a persistent hemothorax that was not adequately drained by the chest tube. In this case, video-assisted thoracoscopy should be considered to evacuate the remaining clot. This procedure reduces the likelihood that a fibrothorax will cause a trapped lung or empyema. It should be performed early (within 7 days). After this point, the fibrin deposits become densely adherent, and their removal is tedious. In general, a small hemothorax can be left alone to reabsorb, but larger ones (estimated at >300 mL radiographically) should be drained. This point is somewhat controversial.

VI Mesothelioma

A. GENERAL CHARACTERISTICS
1. Mesothelioma is the most common primary tumor of the pleura.
2. It is strongly associated with asbestos exposure.
3. It may be diffuse (usually malignant) or localized (often benign). Diffuse mesothelioma spreads along the pleural surface and encompasses the entire lung. These tumors metastasize to the liver, lung, brain, and adrenal glands.
4. It usually occurs in the sixth and seventh decades.

B. CLINICAL FEATURES include:
1. Chest pain
2. Dyspnea
3. Cough
4. Weight loss

C. DIAGNOSIS
1. Chest radiography shows pleural thickening and often a pleural effusion.
2. Chest CT scan identifies metastatic disease as well as the extent and degree of lung and chest wall involvement.
3. Analysis of the pleural fluid may be nondiagnostic.
4. Pleural biopsy performed with thoracoscopy or minithoracotomy is of greater diagnostic value than analysis of pleural fluid.

D. TREATMENT
1. The prognosis is poor despite therapy. Survival after diagnosis is rarely longer than 2 years.
2. When disease is isolated to the ipsilateral hemithorax without lymph node metastasis, radical pleuropneumonectomy may prolong survival. However, the operative mortality rate is high.
3. Neither radiation nor chemotherapy prolongs survival.

Chapter 14

Disorders of the Vascular System

Ⅰ Diabetic Foot

A. GENERAL CHARACTERISTICS

1. Diabetic foot is the development of foot ulcer or gangrene in a patient who has long-standing diabetes.
2. Neurologic, vascular, and architectural changes in the foot lead to the destructive process and increased susceptibility to infection.
3. Thickening of the basement membrane and increased transmural and calcium deposition in the medium and small vessels give rise to stenosis and occlusion of the runoff vessels (distal to the popliteal artery). More proximal vascular involvement is typically less progressive.
4. Infection may range from cellulitis to purulent ulcer to gangrene.
5. Infections are often polymicrobial. They include *Staphylococcus*, *Streptococcus*, *Bacteroides*, and *Clostridia* species.

B. CLINICAL FEATURES

1. Posterior tibial and dorsalis pedis pulses may be present.
2. Dependent rubor or pallor on elevation indicates severe vascular insufficiency to the lower extremity.
3. The ankle–brachial index (ABI) is often normal (>1) or elevated because of extensive mural calcification of the runoff vessels.
4. Ischemic ulcers may occur on the lateral side of the foot, on the toes, or in the web spaces. Tissue necrosis is seen on the heel and malleolar prominences. Neuropathic ulcers arise over the metatarsophalangeal joints.
5. Progressive neuropathy leads to diminished sensation in the foot.

C. DIAGNOSIS

1. Toe pressures measured with **color flow Doppler** are often low because of significant distal vessel disease.
2. When vascular reconstruction is indicated, **arteriography** is required to plan the appropriate procedure.
3. **Magnetic resonance angiography** can be used in patients who have significant renal impairment that may be worsened with angiographic contrast.

D. TREATMENT

1. Conservative therapy first focuses on prevention with adequate foot hygiene and protection with adequate shoes.
2. Callous ulcers on the plantar aspect are debrided daily. For noninfected ulcers, avoidance of weight bearing on the foot prevents repeated trauma and facilitates healing.

3. Infected ulcers must be cleaned. If ischemia occurs, adequate debridement and opening of abscesses must be performed aggressively.

4. Broad-spectrum antibiotics are given initially because many of these infections are polymicrobial. A reasonable combination is ampicillin, gentamicin, and metronidazole. After cultures are done to establish a causative organism, antibiotics are tailored appropriately.

5. Infected bone often requires amputation, as does progressive infection, despite adequate antibiotics and debridement.

6. A demonstrable vascular lesion that impairs blood flow to the foot should be repaired with either angioplasty (short segmental narrowing) or bypass. A reduced ABI (<0.7) usually indicates a significant vascular lesion. Repair is required to facilitate ulcer healing.

Lower Extremity Vascular Occlusive Disease

Lower extremity vascular occlusive disease may be caused by lesions in the femoropopliteal arterial segment or the tibioperoneal segment. Some patients have disease in both areas. The degree of disease and its effect on arterial blood flow to the foot dictate the need, timing, and type of surgical therapy.

A. GENERAL CHARACTERISTICS

1. Vascular occlusive disease in the lower extremities usually results from atherosclerosis.
2. Symptoms progress slowly over time. Only 20%–30% of patients require intervention.
3. The incidence is higher in patients who are older than 50 years of age and have insulin-dependent diabetes.
4. Acute limb ischemia (over hours) is usually embolic rather than the result of progressive vascular disease (over months to years).

B. CLINICAL FEATURES

1. Patients report pain in the calf after walking a specific distance. The pain resolves with rest. Patients who have more severe disease may have foot pain at rest that is worsened with leg elevation.
2. Signs of chronic ischemia to the foot include absence of hair on the toes, dry skin, pallor, dependent rubor, abnormal nail growth, and poor capillary refill (>3 seconds).
3. The femoral pulse is palpable if no proximal arterial occlusion exists. Absent popliteal pulses indicate femoropopliteal disease. The presence of popliteal pulses in the absence of pedal pulses suggests disease in the posterior tibial or dorsalis pedis artery.
4. Nonhealing foot ulcers indicate more severe ischemia. The ulcers may become secondarily infected.

C. DIAGNOSIS

1. **Handheld Doppler** signals that show normal femoral and reduced popliteal signals indicate femoropopliteal artery disease. Normal popliteal signals with diminished posterior tibial or dorsalis pedis signals indicate disease in these respective arteries. The ABI indicates the severity of occlusion. In patients who have severely calcified vessels, the ABI may be normal (>1) because of the noncompressibility of these vessels. This is typically seen in patients with diabetes.
2. An ABI of less than 0.4 indicates limb-threatening ischemia. Symptoms usually begin when the ABI is less than 0.7.
3. **Color flow Doppler** can estimate the degree and location of stenosis. In patients who have noncompressible vessels, toe perfusion pressures are useful in determining the severity of ischemia. Toe pressures of less than 30 mm Hg indicate severe ischemia.

4. Patients who have disabling claudication or rest pain and those who have nonhealing ulcers should undergo color flow Doppler to confirm vascular insufficiency. Doppler also localizes the diseased arterial segments that reduce blood flow. Arteriography of the lower extremity should be performed to provide a road map for surgical bypass or angioplasty. This technique identifies stenosis in the femoropopliteal or tibioperoneal vessels (Figure 14-1).

D. TREATMENT

1. **Nonoperative therapy** can be used with most patients who have intermittent claudication.

    a. **Exercise.** Walking past the point of ischemic symptoms stimulates collateral formation and improves symptoms.

    b. **Smoking.** Cessation of smoking often improves walking distance by more than 100%.

    c. **Medications**

        i. **Pentoxifylline** is a rheologic agent that improves cellular deformability and reduces cellular aggregation to improve flow in the microcirculation. It is clinically proven to improve walking distances.

        ii. **Ticlopidine** is an antiplatelet agent that improves walking distance and ABI.

2. **Operative therapy**

    a. **Indications.** Patients are considered for operative intervention if they have ischemic rest pain, ischemic ulceration, or gangrene. Objectively, patients with an ABI of less than 0.4 or toe perfusion pressures of less than 30 mm Hg have limb-threatening ischemia and should be considered for operative intervention.

    b. **Angioplasty.** Balloon angioplasty is effective in patients who have a short segment of stenosis (usually <3 cm). Most patients have long or multiple segments of superficial femoral artery disease, so this modality is infrequently useful. The most beneficial application is in patients who have poor iliac inflow to the lower extremity with coexistent distal vessel disease that requires a distal bypass. Balloon angioplasty of the stenotic iliac artery is usually effective in improving inflow and graft patency.

    c. **Bypass graft** (Figure 14-2)

        i. A graft is made from the common femoral artery to the popliteal artery above the knee. This graft bypasses the diseased segments in the superficial femoral artery and improves distal flow, provided there is minimal arterial disease in the distal vessels.

        ii. The graft can be formed with a polytetrafluoroethylene (PTFE) tube graft or a vein graft. The 5-year patency rates for saphenous vein grafts are slightly better than that for PTFE (70% vs 60%). Most patients have a previous coronary artery bypass graft and may not have sufficient saphenous vein to permit bypass grafting. PTFE grafts should not be used below the knee because their patency rates are poor. Saphenous vein grafts can be used to create a bypass from the common femoral artery to the posterior tibial artery or the dorsalis pedis artery. The vein must be reversed to allow blood to flow past its valves. If the vein is left in situ, the valves must be lysed with an intraluminal valvulotome. The branches of the vein must also be ligated so that they do not siphon arterial flow distally.

        iii. Warfarin (Coumadin) may be used postoperatively in patients who have poor distal runoff (atherosclerosis of the recipient vessel). No randomized trials show that anticoagulation improves patency, but several reports suggest this effect.

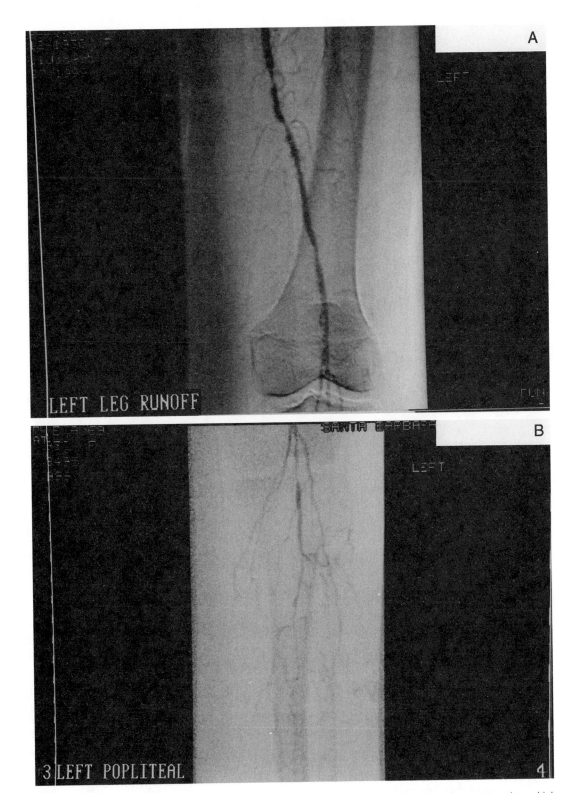

● **Figure 14.1** Angiogram showing (*A*) femoropopliteal and (*B*) tibioperoneal arterial occlusive disease. Note the multiple areas of stenosis.

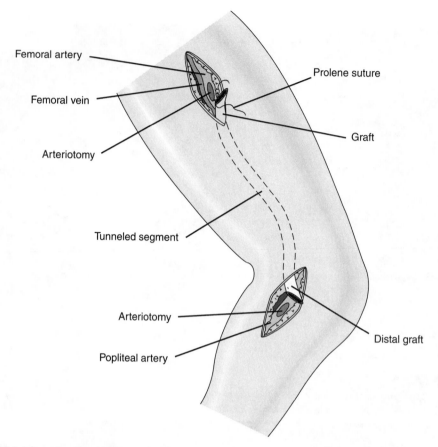

● **Figure 14.2** A femoropopliteal bypass graft showing the proximal and distal anastomoses.

    iv. Follow-up of bypass grafts is important. Repairing a graft before it has completely thrombosed is associated with a higher limb salvage rate than repairing the graft after it has thrombosed. Thrombosis is most likely to occur in the first year after graft placement. The recommended surveillance starts with a duplex of the graft at 1 month after operation, then every 3 months for the first year, every 6 months in the second year, and then yearly.

III Renovascular Hypertension

A. GENERAL CHARACTERISTICS
1. In 5% of patients with hypertension, renovascular hypertension is the cause.
2. Renal artery atherosclerosis is responsible for more than 70% of cases.
3. The remaining cases are caused by fibromuscular dysplasia, which is more common in young women. The intima, media, or adventitia may be involved. The media is the most commonly involved layer in fibromuscular dysplasia. The disease is usually bilateral. However, in unilateral cases, the right renal artery is typically affected.
4. Hypertension is caused by decreased renal perfusion that leads to stimulation of the renin-angiotensin-aldosterone axis.

B. CLINICAL FEATURES
1. Hypertension in a young patient suggests renovascular hypertension.
2. An epigastric bruit may be audible.

   3. Hypertension that is refractory to medical therapy or that requires multiple medications is often reported.

C. DIAGNOSIS

   1. Renal artery duplex scanning is a useful screening test in detecting renal artery stenosis. Stenosis is identified when peak systolic velocity is greater than 180 cm/sec.

   2. Isotope renography is also used to estimate renal blood flow and function. However, it is less sensitive than ultrasound.

   3. Patients whose **ultrasound** findings suggest stenosis should undergo angiography if they have no significant impairment in renal function that could be worsened by iodinated contrast material. **Angiography** identifies the location and nature of the stenosis (Figure 14-3).

   4. Gadolinium-enhanced magnetic resonance angiography can be used in place of conventional angiography if nephrotoxicity is a concern.

D. TREATMENT

   1. Medical therapy is less effective and is associated with a lower long-term survival rate than surgical therapy.

   2. Percutaneous angioplasty is useful in specific cases, including atherosclerotic lesions distal to the renal artery orifice and fibromuscular dysplasia limited to the main renal artery. Lesions located at the orifice are not amenable to angioplasty.

   3. Aortorenal bypass with a reversed saphenous vein graft or PTFE can be performed. In children, vein grafts often become aneurysmal. Therefore, a hypogastric artery graft is used. Renal artery endarterectomy may be useful in treating focal stenosis at the orifice, obviating the need for bypass.

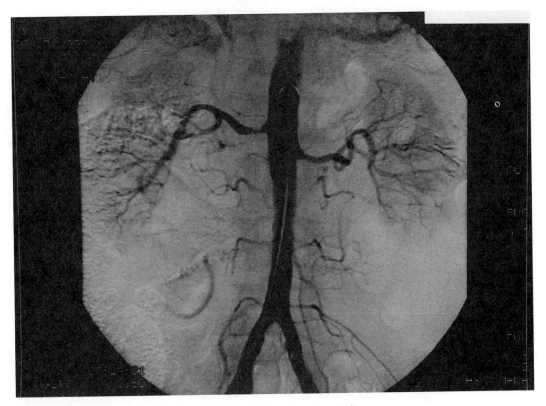

● **Figure 14.3** Angiogram of renal artery stenosis caused by atherosclerotic disease.

Aortic Disease

Abdominal aortic aneurysm (AAA) and aortoiliac occlusive disease are considered here.

A. AAA

  1. General characteristics

    a. The incidence increases with age. AAA occurs in 2%–6% of individuals older than 60 years of age.

    b. The aorta is aneurysmal when its diameter is focally increased by more than 50% of the normal diameter (usually >3 cm).

    c. The most common site of aneurysm formation is in the infrarenal aortic segment.

    d. Coronary artery disease and cerebrovascular disease are often coexistent. These entities must be sought before operative intervention takes place.

    e. The most important predictor of aneurysm rupture is aneurysm size.

  2. Clinical features

    a. Typically, AAAs are asymptomatic and are found incidentally on physical examination as a pulsatile abdominal mass. An abdominal bruit may be audible.

    b. Severe back, flank, or abdominal pain indicates acute expansion, leak, or rupture.

    c. Tachycardia, hypotension, and peritonitis in a patient with a known AAA are likely the result of rupture.

    d. Less commonly, peripheral emboli to the lower extremities may result from dislodged atherosclerotic plaque from the aneurysm wall. The result is an ischemic limb, foot, or toe, depending on the site of embolization.

  3. Diagnosis

    a. Ultrasound is nearly 100% sensitive in detecting AAA. Further, it does not require radiation exposure or intravenous contrast. The study may be less effective in obese patients and those with excessive bowel gas. Clinically, ultrasound is best used to follow an aneurysm, but it should not be used when surgery is contemplated because the proximal and distal extents are poorly identified in relation to the renal and iliac arteries.

    b. Spiral computed tomography (CT) scan with three-dimensional reconstruction provides information about the aneurysm in relation to other structures.

    c. Aortography is used less often with the improved CT scan reconstructions. Its use is of particular significance when specific anatomic detail of the juxtarenal segment is in question or if the patient is being considered for endovascular graft repair.

    d. Patients who have a known or suspected aneurysm as well as shock and peritonitis should not undergo diagnostic evaluation. They require prompt surgical evaluation.

  4. Treatment

    a. Aneurysms smaller than 4 cm are unlikely to rupture. They should be followed annually with CT scan or ultrasound. Aneurysms larger than 5 cm are associated with rupture rates of 30%–40% over 5 years. These patients should be considered for operative repair. Patients who have significant comorbidities and are at significant operative risk may be observed despite an aneurysm of 5 cm. However, when the aneurysm is larger than 8 cm, the risk of rupture is more than 80%. This risk outweighs the operative risk in most patients who have significant comorbidities. The management of patients who have aneurysms 4–5 cm is controversial and must be weighed against the operative risk.

    b. Operative repair may be undertaken with an intraperitoneal or retroperitoneal approach. The retroperitoneal approach is useful in aneurysms that extend to the suprarenal segment. With the retroperitoneal approach, it is difficult to assess the right renal artery and obtain access to the right internal and external iliac arteries.

c. Proximal and distal control of the aorta and iliac vessels above and below the aneurysm is achieved, and the patient is heparinized with 100 U/kg to prevent intravascular clot formation during clamping. The proximal anastomosis is performed after the aneurysm is opened and the plaque is removed. The distal anastomosis is performed to the distal aorta, provided that there is adequate outflow in the iliac arteries. If significant iliac atherosclerosis exists, an aortobifemoral graft can be performed.

d. Patients who have a ruptured AAA need emergent surgical repair without delay for diagnostic tests. In this case, the operative mortality rate is greater than 50%. If the rupture is contained, it may be possible to stabilize the patient on the operating table before incision. This is an important maneuver because in the unstable patient, opening the abdomen results in loss of its tamponade effect and causes further decompensation. If attempts at resuscitation do not reverse the shock, the operation must proceed.

e. Endovascular graft placement was recently used in patients with significant operative risk. The aneurysm must be infrarenal, with a 2-cm proximal neck, to permit proper deployment. If the aneurysm extends to the bifurcation, a bifurcated graft may be used. Long-term studies are under way to evaluate the stability of this form of repair.

f. Operative complications include myocardial infarction (5%), renal insufficiency (6%), hemorrhage (4%), colonic ischemia (5%), impotence (5%–10%), graft infection (1%), and aortoenteric fistula (1%).

B. AORTOILIAC OCCLUSIVE DISEASE

1. General characteristics

a. Atherosclerotic lesions of the aortoiliac vessels usually occur diffusely along the aortoiliac arteries that extend to the infrainguinal common femoral arteries. Less commonly, lesions are limited to the aorta, common iliac vessel, and external iliac vessel. Lesions confined to the terminal aorta and common iliac vessels are least common.

b. Symptoms typically develop during the fifth decade.

2. Clinical features

a. The initial symptoms are associated with exercise. Patients may have intermittent claudication in the buttocks, hips, or thighs. Pain in the calves usually occurs when there is concomitant distal vascular occlusive disease.

b. Men may report impotence with impaired internal iliac artery perfusion.

c. **Leriche's syndrome** (the combination of aortoiliac occlusion or stenosis with hip, buttock, and thigh claudication; impotence; and diminished femoral pulses) may occur.

d. Limb-threatening ischemia usually does not occur unless the patient has associated distal vessel disease or emboli to the distal vessels from the atherosclerotic aortoiliac plaque. Distal emboli may lodge as low as in the small vessels of the toes, leading to gangrene.

e. Some patients have normal femoral pulses at rest because of collateral circulation. However, when examined after exercise, the femoral pulses are typically diminished.

3. Diagnosis

a. For patients who have claudication, the diagnosis may be established with **color duplex ultrasound**. This accurate and noninvasive test shows diminished femoral velocities. This finding indicates an inflow problem.

b. **Angiography** is used for patients who have progressive incapacitating symptoms, rest pain, or limb-threatening ischemia. It may show narrowing of the aorta, common iliac vessels, or internal and external iliac vessels (Figure 14-4).

c. Magnetic resonance angiography may be used in patients who have renal insufficiency. This technique obviates the need for exposure to the nephrotoxicity that is associated with iodine-based intravenous contrast used in conventional angiography.

4. **Treatment**

a. Patients who have claudication without limb-threatening ischemia can be managed nonoperatively with an exercise program and modification of risk factors (e.g., cholesterol-lowering agents, cessation of smoking). Pentoxifylline may be used as a rheologic agent to facilitate arterial flow.

b. Patients who have evidence of embolization to a named distal vessel should undergo prompt embolectomy. Ischemia times greater than 6 hours may lead to irreversible ischemia and limb loss.

c. Short, focal lesions of the iliac arteries are ideally suited for percutaneous angioplasty. This technique obviates the need for surgery and general anesthesia.

d. **Operative management**

i. **Aortobifemoral bypass** is the most commonly used operation. It is indicated for patients who have incapacitating symptoms or limb-threatening ischemia. Perioperative mortality rates are approximately 1%–2%. The 5-year patency rates approach 90%.

ii. **Aortoiliac endarterectomy** is used less often. Its use is restricted to patients who have disease confined to the aorta and common iliac arteries. The

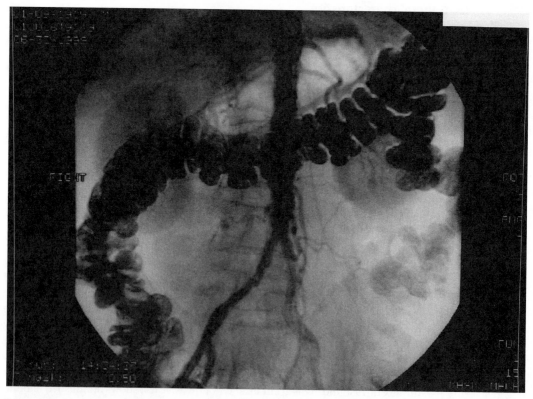

● **Figure 14.4** Angiogram showing aortoiliac arterial occlusive disease.

5-year patency rates are comparable to those with aortobifemoral bypass grafting.

   iii. **Aortoiliac bypass** is less effective for occlusive disease because distal arterial repair of atherosclerotic disease is often needed postoperatively. This procedure is best suited for AAA.

   iv. **Femorofemoral bypass** is useful in treating unilateral iliac disease. This procedure can be performed without general anesthesia (Figure 14-5).

   v. **Axillofemoral bypass** can be used in high-risk surgical patients. A femorofemoral bypass can be added if bilateral iliac disease is present. Patency results are variable.

Ⓥ Carotid Artery Occlusive Disease

A. GENERAL CHARACTERISTICS

1. Stroke is usually caused by internal carotid atherosclerotic disease with embolization to distal intracerebral vessels. Cerebral ischemia may also be caused by a low-flow state.

2. The carotid bifurcation is typically the site of disease because of the turbulent flow generated at this site. The enlarging plaque may ulcerate and hemorrhage within itself, and may cause thrombosis or embolization.

3. Asymptomatic patients often have carotid artery disease that is detected during evaluation for other procedures (e.g., coronary artery bypass, aortic aneurysm repair).

4. The risk of stroke in the first year after a transient ischemic attack is 10%–30%. The cumulative risk of stroke in the subsequent 5 years is 30%–50%.

5. The risk of stroke in patients who have asymptomatic carotid disease increases with increasing stenosis. Stenosis greater than 75% is associated with a stroke risk of 20%–40%.

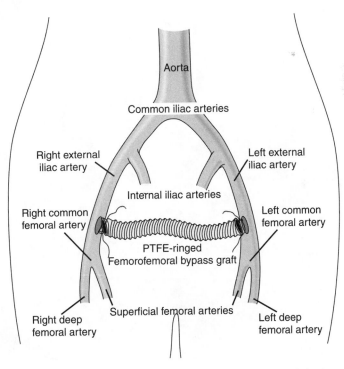

● **Figure 14.5** A femorofemoral bypass graft with polytetrafluoroethylene (*PTFE*) tunneled subcutaneously.

B. CLINICAL FEATURES

1. A **transient ischemic attack (TIA)** is a focal neurologic deficit that develops and resolves within 24 hours. TIAs may cause weakness and sensory loss contralateral to the side of the diseased carotid vessel.
2. **Transient monocular blindness** may occur ipsilateral to the diseased carotid vessel.
3. **Stroke** is caused by permanent cerebral infarction that leads to a permanent neurologic deficit.
4. **Carotid bruit** may be present, but its absence does not preclude carotid artery disease.

C. DIAGNOSIS

1. **Color flow duplex** identifies the degree of carotid stenosis. It can be used as the sole preoperative diagnostic modality before carotid endarterectomy. If the duplex scan suggests complete occlusion, an **angiogram** may be indicated to ensure that complete occlusion is present.
2. **Angiography** is the gold standard for identifying carotid artery atherosclerosis and determining its extent. Arteriography is associated with a stroke rate of 2%–4% as well as nephrotoxicity. Therefore, its use is decreasing (Figure 14-6).
3. **Magnetic resonance angiography** is noninvasive and provides similar visualization without risk. If a duplex scan is equivocal or indicates complete occlusion, this modality may be used instead of angiography.
4. In a patient who has had an acute stroke, **CT scan** of the brain is necessary to document the area involved and to distinguish between hemorrhagic and infarcted stroke.

D. TREATMENT

1. **Medical management** includes control of hypertension, cessation of smoking, use of cholesterol-lowering agents, and exercise. Anticoagulation and aspirin do not sig-

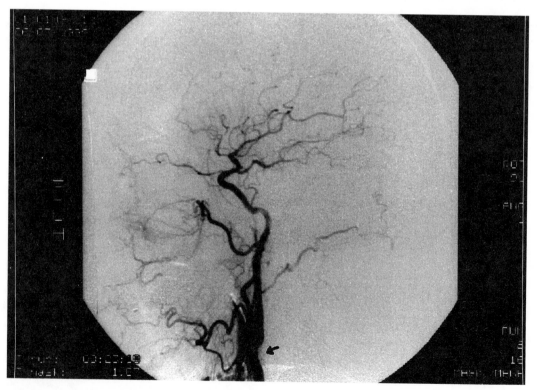

● **Figure 14.6** Angiogram showing internal carotid artery stenosis.

nificantly reduce stroke risk. Aspirin can reduce the mortality rate by lowering the risk of myocardial infarction in patients who have coexistent coronary artery disease.

2. Indications for **carotid artery endarterectomy** include TIA, stroke with minimal residual deficit, and high-grade stenosis (typically >75%). Carotid endarterectomy involves proximal and distal control of the common carotid, external, internal, and superior thyroid arteries. After heparinization with 100 U/kg, the vessels are clamped. The carotid vessel is opened from the bifurcation and along the internal carotid artery. A shunt from the common carotid artery to the distal internal carotid artery may be used. The plaque is removed, and the arteriotomy is closed (Figure 14-7).

3. Stroke may occur perioperatively as a result of inadequate collateral blood flow during carotid occlusion, embolization during dissection, occlusion from an intimal flap at the endarterectomy end point, or embolization from a platelet aggregate on the surface of the endarterectomized artery. As a result, patients who awaken from carotid endarterectomy with a stroke must undergo prompt reexploration to exclude an intimal flap or platelet aggregate that can be remedied. The operative stroke risk is approximately 3%.

4. Recurrent stenosis within 6 months of surgery is usually caused by intimal hyperplasia. Restenosis after 2 years or longer is caused by atherosclerotic disease.

5. Perioperative blood pressure control is imperative to reduce the risk of hemorrhagic stroke and reduce myocardial oxygen demands.

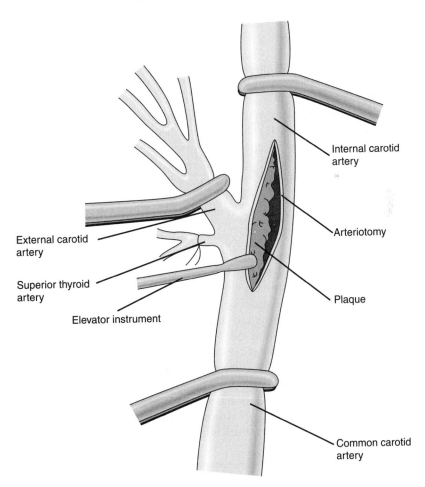

● **Figure 14.7** Carotid endarterectomy showing the carotid arteriotomy and plaque removal.

6. Preoperative cardiac workup is indicated only for patients who have significant angina or dysrhythmia.

VI Venous Insufficiency (Varicose Veins)

A. GENERAL CHARACTERISTICS
1. Venous insufficiency affects as many as 25% of the general population.
2. Chronic elevation in venous pressure results from valvular insufficiency of the superficial or deep venous system. It may also occur as a result of venous thrombosis.
3. Venous insufficiency usually develops after the fourth decade or during pregnancy.
4. The prevalence is increased among people with occupations that involve long periods of standing and among those with a family history.

B. CLINICAL FEATURES
1. Dilated, tortuous, easily compressible superficial veins in the lower extremity indicate venous insufficiency.
2. Varicosities over the medial thigh and lower leg are caused by greater saphenous insufficiency. Lesser saphenous incompetence results in posterior calf varicosities.
3. Aching and itching are common and are increased at the end of the day. Relief is achieved by elevating the leg.
4. Brown pigmentation over the medial perimalleolar region results from increased deposition of fibrin and hemosiderin in the subcutaneous tissues as a result of elevated venous pressure. Fibrosis develops and leads to lipodermatosclerosis.
5. Prolonged insufficiency leads to ankle edema and venous stasis ulcers over the medial perimalleolar area. Cellulitis may occur around the ulcer.

C. DIAGNOSIS
1. A **handheld Doppler** can identify incompetent valves at the femoral level by noting retrograde signals during the Valsalva maneuver. Similarly, when the patient is standing and the leg is squeezed, flow toward the heart is heard. However, when the leg is released, a retrograde signal indicates valvular insufficiency above the position of the handheld Doppler.
2. **Duplex ultrasound** provides additional information by identifying venous obstruction, incompetent valves, or incompetent perforating veins.

D. TREATMENT
1. If varicosities are present, but there is no insufficiency at the saphenofemoral junction, **sclerotherapy** may be used to obliterate the varicosities. A concentrated sodium chloride solution can be injected directly into the varicosity in the office setting.
2. Saphenofemoral incompetence requires **saphenous vein stripping** and **ligation** at the saphenofemoral junction. Individual varicosities are then ligated or stripped through small stab wound incisions.
3. Venous ulcer, or lipodermatosclerosis, is often associated with an underlying perforating vein. Ligation of this vein permits healing of the involved area and is a useful adjunct to local wound therapy for recurring venous stasis ulcers.
4. Healing of venous stasis ulcers is often accomplished by an occlusive dressing that diminishes ankle edema. This is most often accomplished with an Unna boot. If infection or cellulitis is present, antibiotics are required to cover gram-positive organisms (e.g., ampicillin).
5. Patients with destruction of valves or elongated floppy valves may benefit from vein valve transplant with an axillary vein that bears a valve or from vein valvuloplasty, respectively.

VII Deep Venous Thrombosis (DVT)

A. GENERAL CHARACTERISTICS

1. Thrombosis in the deep venous system of the lower extremities and iliac veins results from changes in the venous walls, stasis, and a hypercoagulable state (Virchow's triad).
2. Other risk factors include obesity, malignancy, trauma, immobility, age older than 40 years, pregnancy, protein C deficiency, protein S deficiency, and antithrombin III deficiency.
3. General anesthesia is believed to promote venous thrombosis through venodilation, which disrupts the endothelial lining and exposes the thrombogenic endothelial surface.
4. Detection of DVT is critical because of the risk of subsequent pulmonary embolism, which carries a significant risk of mortality.

B. CLINICAL FEATURES

1. Fever of unknown origin should prompt a search for DVT.
2. Lower extremity edema and pain with dorsiflexion of the foot (Homans' sign) is seen in fewer than 30% of cases.

C. DIAGNOSIS

1. **Color flow Doppler** is the diagnostic modality of choice. It is highly accurate in detecting lower extremity clots. Nonocclusive clots in the iliac veins are less accurately detected because they cannot be visualized. If the thrombus does not cause flow changes, the color flow Doppler will not detect a clot.
2. Other modalities that are less commonly used include radioactive iodine-labeled fibrinogen and impedence plethysmography.

D. TREATMENT

1. Prophylaxis involves improving venous circulation in the lower extremities before induction of anesthesia. Sequential compression stockings are used for this purpose. These devices stimulate the release of fibrinolytic products that also may provide some benefit. Therefore, some prophylaxis may be achieved by placing these devices on the upper extremities.
2. Prophylactic low-dose heparin (5000 U subcutaneously every 8–12 hours) is effective in reducing pulmonary embolus by 50% and DVT by 60%–70%. It is associated with minor bleeding complications in up to 2% of patients. Similarly, in orthopedic studies, new low–molecular-weight heparin showed slightly better results in DVT prevention with slightly fewer bleeding complications.
3. Once DVT is detected, systemic anticoagulation is initiated with the goal of prolonging the partial thromboplastin time to twice normal. This typically requires an initial bolus of 100–150 U/kg intravenously followed by a maintenance infusion starting at 17 U/kg/hr. Oral anticoagulation is then started with Coumadin to prolong the international normalized ratio to 2.0–3.0. Once this ratio is achieved, heparinization can be discontinued. Coumadin is continued for 3–6 months.
4. If anticoagulation is contraindicated, or if a pulmonary embolus develops despite anticoagulation therapy, then the placement of a vena cava filter is indicated to prevent pulmonary embolus.

Index

Page numbers in *italics* denote figures; those followed by a t denote tables.